THE
POWER
OF
SELF-
HEALING

Take Action Over Your Trauma

THE
POWER
OF
SELF-
HEALING

Dr Sarah Woodhouse
TRAUMA EXPERT & COACHING PSYCHOLOGIST

GREEN TREE

LONDON · OXFORD · NEW YORK · NEW DELHI · SYDNEY

GREEN TREE
Bloomsbury Publishing Plc
50 Bedford Square, London, WC1B 3DP, UK
Bloomsbury Publishing Ireland Limited
29 Earlsfort Terrace, Dublin 2, D02 AY28, Ireland

BLOOMSBURY, GREEN TREE and the Green Tree logo are
trademarks of Bloomsbury Publishing Plc

First published in Great Britain 2025

A catalogue record for this book is available from the British Library

Library of Congress Cataloguing-in-Publication data has been applied for

ISBN: HB: 978-1-3994-2439-4; eBook: 978-1-3994-2434-9

2 4 6 8 10 9 7 5 3 1

Typeset in ITC Berkeley Oldstyle by Midland Typesetters, Australia
Printed and bound in Great Britain by Clays Ltd, Elcograf S.p.A.

To find out more about our authors and books visit www.bloomsbury.com
and sign up for our newsletters
For product safety related questions contact productsafety@bloomsbury.com

This book is for my clients, literally.

In particular I'd like to thank Lucy, Harriette,
Naomi, Helen, Claudette and Rose.

Your self-led action and courage have inspired this book.

Thank you x

Contents

Introduction

In this book I'm going to show you how to heal your trauma and create real change in yourself, your relationships and your life. And, even better, I'm going to show you that you don't need therapy to achieve these things.

I'm not anti-therapy, I'm just pro-you. *You* waking up, taking action, reconnecting to your adult self and unlocking your own power to heal your trauma. This message can be easily (and lazily) spun to make me sound like the bad guy. So I'm going to say it again: I'm not anti-therapy.

I'm not anti-therapy, but I have come to understand that therapy alone cannot heal childhood trauma. I understand this because of my profession *and* because of my personal experience. I spent decades in therapy and did *not* heal my trauma. Despite all the talking, all the different therapists, all the intentions and all the learning, I did not do the one thing I needed to do to truly heal. And that *thing* that I did not do is what this book is about. It's the secret no-one tells us. It's the most important, empowering, liberating and terrifying thing you will ever learn about wellness and thriving. It's the non-negotiable, blindingly-obvious-once-you-know-it truth of trauma healing. The truth is: *you* have the power to heal your trauma, but to heal, you must take action. Therapy alone cannot heal trauma, but therapy coupled with structured and meaningful self-led action will create profound, deep healing and trans-formation. Because as we take action, we break free from old trauma-led patterns and develop a whole new way of being and relating.

This truth becomes self-evident and indisputable once we understand what trauma actually does. Childhood trauma, or any trauma in fact, creates an incomplete nervous system response to a perceived threat. We quite literally get stuck in fight, flight, freeze, fawn or collapse. What's happening in our nervous system shapes our thinking, our behaviour, our body, our emotions, our identity and sense of self, and our ways of coping. It affects how we relate to ourselves and others. It affects how we live. It affects *everything*. This is particularly true for those of us with *childhood* trauma because the patterns of behaviour, led by the nervous system response, are so deeply ingrained. We've been unconsciously practising these patterns (such as anxiety, avoidance, people-pleasing, compulsive over-thinking and worrying) since we were children. Childhood trauma is also referred to as developmental trauma, which is a wholly accurate term, as trauma experienced from birth to the age of 18 affects how we develop and grow. Healing then, necessarily, requires us to learn a new way of relating and living. It is an un-learning, an un-doing and a re-patterning. And no matter how good our therapist, coach, psycholo-gist or practitioner might be, we cannot sit in a room for an hour a week and learn *a whole new way of being*. To do this, we must take empowered action during the other 167 hours a week. To heal our dysregulated, traumatised mind, body and sense of self we must act, not just talk about acting. We must act, not just think about acting. We must act.

The sad truth is that our expert-led mental health system can induce in us a sense of dependence and disempowerment. We can easily and quickly feel as though we have little agency and are not in control of our own healing. I believe this is one of the key reasons I didn't get well sooner. I'd outsourced my agency and my power. I put my therapist on a pedestal. I put *all* therapists on a pedestal. My childhood trauma whispered to me: 'You're getting this wrong, they all know more.' I was searching, hypervigilantly looking for the best therapist, the best practitioner who would bless me with their 'better-than-me-ness'. I was looking for the answer outside of myself. I believed that I couldn't effect change and that I needed someone else to fix me.

I believed this because I had unresolved childhood trauma (which strips us of our agency and leaves us in a state of freeze and powerlessness), yes. But also because it's what I had been overtly and covertly taught by society. I had been taught, both professionally and personally, that trauma was complex and extremely specialised, and therefore belonged to the clinical and medical domain. That I needed someone (probably a man) with a great many qualifications to *fix* me. That trauma healing was elusive and hard to attain, rather than readily available within me.

The message in this book is simple but radical: trauma healing is far from elusive. It's a very real thing we can all learn, implement and attain as we reclaim our agency and power by taking daily action. And I'll show you how, step by step.

Everything required to heal your trauma exists within you right now. Literally, everything. But to access your own power to create deep healing, you must become willing to practise and experience a new way of being and relating. No-one told you this before now because they know how terrifying this truth can be. This truth means we must stop looking to others to heal us and instead start to take responsibility for our own healing. It means we must accept we are more powerful than our trauma led us to believe. We must also do the one thing we've been subconsciously avoiding: change. And as intoxicating and appealing as *change* first sounds, really, truly, deeply changing is quite literally the scariest thing any human with trauma can attempt to do.

Fame and fortune are readily bestowed on humans who tell other humans what they want to hear. So I'm taking a risk here. You might not want to hear what I'm going to say because I'm going to talk about personal responsibility, daily action and real change. The approach I'm going to teach you is far from an intoxicating 'heal in a weekend' one. I know we'd all prefer a magic pill. I'd much rather take two 'cure childhood trauma pills' every morning over learning a whole new way of being. I know this way is harder. I know it takes effort. I know this because I've been there (searching for a cure outside of myself, hoping that the next therapist is the therapist who will heal me, resisting doing the one thing I actually need to do: take action).

Hopefully my lack of pandering will help you trust me. Because I suspect you know that no one would advocate *this* approach if it wasn't effective.

Trauma exists as an old way of being – an old subconscious playbook that no longer serves us. Trauma healing *emerges* as we learn a new way of being. That may seem like an overwhelmingly large task. But this book breaks it down in an accessible, logical way. You'll come to see that despite the glorious long-term outcomes, we actually achieve this in the short term by repeating (and repeating and repeating) simple daily actions and principles designed to increase and build specific capacities. These *capacities* are currently limited, or entirely missing, because of your trauma.

As well as teaching you how to heal your trauma through self-led action and capacity building, I'm also going to tell you a little bit about how I learned this lesson the hard way. Life kicking my ass has always been my greatest teacher. I write this book not just from the perspective of a trauma specialist, but as a human who was urgently called to heal herself. In a very real way, I've had to practise what I preach. I've road tested everything included in this book, and as I took action, I moved from debilitating collapse and illness into health, well-being and healing.

This approach may not be the magic pill you might want, but I promise you that it's precisely what you need to truly heal.

Childhood trauma

Childhood trauma produces an incomplete nervous system response to a 'perceived threat' that feels overwhelming and insurmountable. *Perceived threats* in childhood can be anything at all that makes a child feel unsafe. If the threat feels overwhelming and insurmountable (i.e. if the child can't respond to it and deal with it) their survival response (fight, flight, freeze, fawn or collapse) will not properly switch off. Given that newborns, infants and children are naturally defenceless and unable to respond, threats can easily feel overwhelming and insurmountable. This means that traumatic reactions in childhood are common and widespread.

Childhood trauma often results from a threat to a child's sense of connection to their parents or carers. In evolutionary terms, this makes sense because children are completely reliant on the adults in their lives, so anything that endangers this bond can feel like a threat to their whole existence. Childhood experiences like emotional neglect, emotional disconnection, harsh parental criticism or shaming, rejection, adoption, divorce, or a physically or mentally unwell parent, can feel *overwhelmingly* threatening to a child. Threats to a child's resources and structural stability (such as financial instability, parental job loss, bankruptcy, having to emigrate or even move house) can also feel overwhelmingly threatening. And, of course, threats to a child's life and body (such as a physical attack, car accident, illness, accidents, physical or sexual abuse) are highly likely to be experienced as deeply overwhelming for a child.

Despite being an uncomfortable read, I hope this overview of common childhood traumatic experiences is helpful. Either way, more important than understanding the cause is understanding the effect (i.e. the traumatic reaction).

You're going to learn that traumatic reactions are painfully broad. As I wrote my first book, *You're Not Broken*, I was keen to help the reader understand that so much of what they experience is part of the ballooning traumatic reaction. Insecure? Trauma. Bad back? Trauma. Chronic fatigue? Trauma. Can't stop shopping? Trauma. There is truth in this message – so much *is* trauma-led. But as I write this book, I also know that stating, 'It's all trauma' can be unhelpful. What we really need are specifics. We need to know where trauma healing begins and ends and where, say, a chiropractor might be helpful. This book is all about the specifics, so I won't go into too much detail here, but suffice to say that survival responses are designed to keep us safe and *away from* threats. Over time, these responses become deeply ingrained and automatic, and negatively affect our mental and physical health, our relationships, our careers and our entire sense of self.

Childhood trauma locks us into unconscious autopilot. Our trauma does not want us to change or deviate from these protective patterns because it does not know the threat has passed. It calls us to stay in patterns of flight, fight, freeze, fawn or collapse because it thinks repeating what's familiar is safe. In its rigidity it strips us of our agency, our power and our choice. It prevents us from healing because healing requires change, flow and flexibility.

You might have heard this idea – that trauma leaves us stuck and repeating old patterns – before. Because everyone is talking about trauma nowadays, right? The thing is, I knew this too. And when I say *knew*, I literally mean I studied it for over a decade. As an academic, I well understood the complex interplay of neural, social and behavioural trauma symptoms. But still, I was unable to see (let alone change) the most insidious and buried trauma-led patterns that were profoundly harming my mind, body and soul.

My new lowest point

Seven years ago I developed weird neurological symptoms. My vision often blurred, my left foot felt weird and tingly, and I felt permanently dizzy and weak. I was deeply afraid because I knew something was terribly wrong. In all honesty, at times I felt sure I was going to die. But here we are seven years later and I'm far from dead. I do, however, have multiple sclerosis

(MS), which I'll admit isn't the, 'Yay, it was all a dream' kind of happy ending I was hoping to manifest.

This part of my story may feel unrelatable. Perhaps you're thinking, 'Ah, no, this book isn't for me – this is written for *other* people, for *sick* people.' Well, I'd ask you to read just a little more, as I suspect it's about to get a lot more relatable.

Two years before the diagnosis I was doing *all* the things. I was setting up a business, working hard, growing my family, planning, creating and striving. From the outside I appeared productive, driven and ambitious. Internally, though, I was chronically stressed, adrenalised, anxious, stuck in my head and disconnected from my body. I was living in survival – oscillating between fight, flight, freeze and fawn. I can describe the me of ten years ago with painful accuracy thanks to three things: time passing, healing and good old-fashioned hindsight. Now I can see the stress and disconnection, but at the time I was disturbingly unaware. On some level I knew I was not okay, but my whole adult identity and life were built around the idea that I was now very okay and very healed. I'd spent 15 years studying trauma as a research psychologist, and decades in therapy, but somehow here I was on autopilot, racing towards an autoimmune diagnosis associated with chronic stress and childhood trauma.

As well as being the worst year of my life, this was also the year I took responsibility for my own healing. I stopped waiting for someone else to fix me and started to heal myself. The diagnosis called me to action, which in turn created deep change and healing. *This* is what had been missing, and *this* is what I dearly want for you too.

There are gifts hidden in any kind of wake-up call. Whether it's a diagnosis like anxiety or depression, a family breakdown, job loss, illness, financial problems, relationship issues, divorce, burnout or any other painful situation, wake-up calls present us with a choice. We can carry on down the same path and face the same outcomes. Or we can courageously try a different, new way. These moments let us in on the secret to trauma healing because they reveal that we need to change.

Before the diagnosis, I was about 30 per cent there on 'doing it differently'. The diagnosis taught me that trauma healing requires a far greater willingness to *do it all differently*. Not just 'a bit different', then. Not just reading a self-help book and doing 20 minutes of yoga a week. Really, truly, radically different. To heal, we have to develop a different way of being, living and relating. We learn to approach our day differently. We learn to talk to ourselves differently. We learn to cope with stress differently. We develop a different relationship with ourselves and our bodies. We learn to connect to others differently and to be in the world differently.

As we make changes and create new habits, we simultaneously return home to our body and to our self. The changes we implement enable connection to an authentic sense of self that feels profoundly true. Oddly, the whole process of doing things differently feels very much like coming home.

Trauma healing is about creating new habits that break old patterns. But to do things differently we have to become consciously (often painfully) aware of the trauma-led patterns we're stuck in. We become aware of these patterns in our thinking, bodies, emotions, behaviour, our beliefs about ourselves and our sense of identity. Conscious awareness of our trauma leads us to create a meaningfully different inner world as well as a meaningfully different outer world.

As I explain it this way, I suppose it sounds relatively simple. But the issue is that the very thing we're trying to see and heal doesn't want to be seen. Trauma operates outside of conscious awareness, sneakily building up sophisticated patterns of protection and survival in a way that we either barely notice or falsely believe we have chosen.

Conscious awareness isn't something we can just click our fingers and have. If we don't take it slowly, the awareness itself can be traumatic. Trust me when I say that 'coming into awareness' (which this book will teach you) is a far gentler option than my approach to waking up, which was, I suppose, a rock-bottom. The diagnosis was a new lowest point following at least two previous new lowest points. It's interesting that so many of us only act once we've been faced with exceptionally painful consequences. That pain is the thing to propel us into real change. I'm really hoping the diagnosis was my final new lowest point. Fingers crossed I'm not writing book three from prison. Although given that my healing seems predicated by me getting metaphorically hit by a bus, who knows.

Truthfully, my new lowest point often felt too much for me to hold and process. Despite this, or perhaps because of this, something important within me shifted. I was humbled, open and willing (even desperate) to learn a new way of being. For one of the first times in my life my fear of change was less potent than my deep need to keep doing things the same way. The scale had tipped. Doing it the way I'd always done it no longer felt appealing, safe or smart because it had helped create the painful consequences I now faced.

The diagnosis snapped me into conscious awareness. And after an appropriate period of blind panic and deep regret, it put a fire in my belly.

'No,' I thought. 'No, this is not my story.'

The diagnosis was the moment I reclaimed my agency and my power. Over that godawful year I went from autopilot – unconsciously reacting and repeating old patterns – to reclaiming my power to create positive change. I went from subconsciously believing I had little choice over how I experience life to understanding that I did have a choice, and that I would (not *could*, but *would*) create real change. In geek terms, this is called post-traumatic growth (PTG), and no matter how stuck you are, I want this spark for you too. By the end of this book you're going to know, deep down in your bones, that you have agency, that you have choices, that you can do things differently, that you can create meaningful, profound change in yourself and your life and that you can heal your trauma.

What I've just written may not sound revolutionary, but it is. Because what I'm saying isn't just reflective of my own story and experience, it's reflective of a fundamental shift in how we approach healing and mental health. For decades, we've collectively dismissed and denied our own ability to create and maintain healing by labelling it 'self-help'. But now there's a very real understanding that we can achieve profound trauma healing outside the clinic room.

The revolution

We're in the middle of a revolution in how we understand and approach mental and physical health. This empowering *shift* has been fuelled by three interwoven developments within the trauma field, which are challenging everything we thought we knew about mental and physical health and how to heal. This shift is still largely being ignored by mainstream medicine, as well as many psychologists. This is to be expected: paradigm shifts in knowledge are uncomfortable and always met with resistance. But there will come a point when no one can deny this growing body of evidence – it's slowly becoming the norm.

The first development is the inclusion of Complex-Posttraumatic Stress Disorder (C-PTSD) in the official psychiatric diagnostic manual, the *International Classification of Diseases (11th Revision)*.[1] In other words, psychiatrists can now diagnose someone with C-PTSD. This is massive because C-PTSD is the mental health condition that can develop if you experience chronic long-term trauma, such as childhood trauma. For decades leading psychotherapists, treatment centres and clued-in psychologists have been treating childhood trauma. But they've been doing so with little official recognition from the mainstream medical-aligned branches of psychology and psychiatry. Now, we're naming it, and I'll say this again: *this* is massive.

Importantly, the diagnostic criteria also clarify the core symptoms of complex trauma, explicitly stating what childhood trauma *is*. The diagnostic manual states that C-PTSD consists of the core symptoms of PTSD (i.e. intrusive thoughts, avoidance behaviours and sense of current threat) *and* includes problems regulating emotions, a sense of worthlessness and difficulty sustaining relationships.[2]

The official stamp of psychiatric approval and the new clarity we have about the core symptoms is validating. You probably didn't need this validation to know that your experience, your pain, your trauma, is real. But it helps. Such validation is all the more important because those with childhood trauma are already predisposed to minimise and deny their pain. We self-blame or we're loyal to the point of self-annihilation. We do this to protect ourselves It can feel safer to blame ourselves than admit that we were treated badly. It's a smart way of coping, really. But the greater recognition of C-PTSD is a tangible, visible sign of the revolution that's occurring – one that acknowledges complex trauma as a very real thing that causes immense pain and dysfunction in our sense of self and relationships.

The second development comes from longitudinal research into the effect of childhood trauma on long-term health. Mounting research demonstrates that adverse childhood experiences (ACEs), such as abuse, neglect and household dysfunction, contribute to long-term health issues.[3] Cardiovascular disease, cancer and respiratory disease are all associated with experiencing multiple different traumas in childhood.[4] So too are autoimmune issues (for example, and this is just off the top of my head, MS).[5] The mechanisms for this causality aren't yet fully understood, but there's broad consensus that systemic toxic stress and inflammation are the main agents.[6] In other words, trauma responses lead to persistently high levels of cortisol and adrenaline in the body, which in turn lead to inflammation and illness.

I find the ACEs research a little depressing, to be honest. Admittedly, maybe that's because I'm already one of these statistics. But I think it's more to do with the fact that it's all so blindingly obvious. I'm irritated that it's taken so long for us to collectively acknowledge that, 'Oh shit, would you look at that, trauma in childhood is really bad for the body.' I find it even more irritating that a considerable proportion of the mainstream medical community remain completely unaware of this fact. Although I should add that a doctor approached me in a café a few weeks ago and asked me to come and explain the links between childhood trauma and physical deterioration to his department at the local hospital. So, you know, maybe it's not all doctors.

This development is also *massive* because it tells a new story about the interconnected nature of the mind and body. This research teaches us that trauma is not *just* emotional, it's also physiological. Healing trauma necessarily involves healing the body by helping our nervous system move out of chronic fight-flight and/or freeze, fawn or collapse.

The third development is the exploding popularity of Polyvagal Theory. The influence of this theory, proposed by Dr Stephen Porges in 1994,[7] is everywhere, even if you don't realise it. It's why you keep reading about the benefits of ice baths and why we're all suddenly into long exhalations and yoga nidra.

In a nutshell, this theory describes how the neural circuits in our autonomic nervous system (ANS) are constantly scanning for signs of safety and signs of threat. This process, which Porges calls *neuroception*, happens outside of conscious awareness. Just as we breathe without telling ourselves to breathe, we constantly scan our internal and external environments for signs of safety and threat without telling ourselves to do so. The theory centres around the role of the vagus nerve in this scanning process, hence the name 'Polyvagal' Theory. The vagus nerve is the main neural component of the parasympathetic nervous system (the part responsible for moving us out of arousal and go-go-go energy and into rest and repair). This nerve is so extensive and meandering that in many ways it *is* the parasympathetic nervous system. The vagus nerve consists of two main parts. The 'ventral' (front) side of the nerve responds to cues of safety in our internal world, environment and relationships. It supports feelings of physical safety and emotional connection to others. When the ventral vagal nerve is operating we feel connected, open, curious, compassionate, present and regulated. The 'dorsal' (back) side of the vagus nerve responds to cues of danger. It pulls us away from connection, out of awareness and into a state of self-protection. In moments when we might experience a cue of danger we can begin to shut down and feel frozen, indicating that our dorsal vagal nerve has taken over. Polyvagal Theory has taught us that an *unconscious* nervous system response shapes our sense of connection to ourselves and others, guides our behaviour and creates our emotional experience.[8]

Polyvagal Theory is wildly complicated, so I'm going to stop now before we all regret starting this. So let me tell you now what this theory means for you. Or rather, let Deb Dana – the practitioner who has made Polyvagal Theory accessible – explain in her own words. She writes that although the autonomic nervous system is shaped by early life experiences, it can also be 'reshaped with ongoing experience, that habitual response patterns can be interrupted, and that new patterns can be created'.[9]

In other words, we can utilise neuroception and reshape our system to pick up on cues of safety. Polyvagal Theory also teaches that small, incremental changes will lead to transformational change first in the nervous system and then in our experience of life. Dana also states that although therapy sessions are useful for discovery and learning, the time between sessions must be used to 'encourage mastery'.

These three developments have combined to demonstrate something new and radically different. To summarise, here's what they collectively tell us:

Childhood trauma is real and damaging. It greatly impacts our sense of self, our beliefs and our relationships. As well as affecting our long-term mental health, living in a near-permanent state of fight-flight-freeze can greatly impact our physical health and potenitally lead to long-term illness, such as cardiovascular disease.[10] Although the nervous system has become locked into patterns of threat-detection and protection, we can slowly move the body out of survival mode and shape the system towards safety and connection.

Just as these developments highlight the role of the nervous system in the devastation that childhood trauma causes, they also reveal the nervous system's power and potential to heal our mind, body *and* our sense of self. The nervous system is capable of nothing short of magic. Just as it moves us into stress and survival in response to signs of threat, we can take action to reshape it to support flourishing, connection and healing.

'We can take action' are the most important words in the previous sentence. We can. *You* can. You can learn simple tools and principles to use daily, and as you take action you can heal your trauma. I know this because I have done it. I've moved from collapse to regulation and thriving. I've also had the privilege of witnessing hundreds of clients create the same change and healing by taking self-led action one day at a time.

I get goosebumps as I write this. Firstly, because it's true, and secondly, because what I'm describing has the potential to change your whole experience of life.

Self-led doesn't mean alone

As I talk about taking action, I need to be very clear that I'm not suggesting you do this alone. Far from it. This call to action is separate to whether you do, or do not, choose to work with a trauma therapist. It's about agency and self-efficacy – your inner belief that *you* can effect positive change in yourself and your life.

I still work with trauma therapists and practitioners. But it's so very different now. Now I know I'm the one doing the work. Now I say what I need. I only work with clinicians who are fully and firmly focused on empowering me. Now I know that as well as showing up for a session, I must also take self-led action in the other 167 hours a week for the healing to integrate. So, my message truly isn't about doing it alone. It's about getting as much support as you need while recognising that to heal you must also take action.

The newer trauma treatments empower clients and encourage self-led healing and mastery. For example, Somatic Experiencing (SE), Somatic Regulation and Resilience (SRR) and Internal Family Systems (IFS) have all combined a nervous system approach with a developmental trauma approach to create empowering modalities that heal clients while also teaching them how to take action to heal themselves. *See pages 109–12, 139, 155–9, 234–45, 316 for more information on these models and other trauma treatment modalities.* These new treatments were born from the three developments in the field I outlined on pages 11–16, and they're changing the therapeutic relationship by creating more equality and collaboration.

Throughout this book you're going to hear from different trauma practitioners. I asked many of them why they think coaching is the second fastest growing global sector[11] and what role it plays in the future of trauma healing. Their answers were fascinating: people want more agency, they want tools, they want to work with the body and nervous system, they want to focus on solutions, they want equality in the relationship with their practitioner. They want to be empowered. They want collaboration. They don't want the traditional model of a 'blank slate' therapist who brings nothing of themselves. They want authentic connection. Coaching is growing exponentially – so much so that many therapists and psychologists now incorporate coaching methods into their approach.

People are increasingly unable to tolerate the 'ivory tower' and, I believe, sense it is perpetuating, rather than deconstructing, systemic trauma.

Change is happening and I'm for it.

When I pitched this book to the publisher I said: 'It's just the right side of controversial – not so controversial I'll be professionally black-listed, but controversial enough to ruffle some feathers.'

They liked this idea very much, so here we are.

Saying that our current outdated mental health systems can strip us of our agency and disempower us isn't outrageous. Saying that trauma healing calls each of us to take action and reclaim our power to self-heal isn't scandalous. But it's also true that these points may not go down well with some clinicians.

I'm not making these points because I want to be controversial for the sake of it. This is my thesis because I know it to be true intellectually and, perhaps more importantly, I believe it with all my heart. More than anything, this is what the MS diagnosis has taught me. And I believe it's time we confidently and collectively acknowledge the revolution and what it means for each of us.

Other voices

The clinicians I've asked to share their expertise are experienced professionals with unique perspectives. More importantly, they've done their own trauma work. As a result, they're balanced, grounded, curious, compassionate, regulated, open-hearted humans. They also share my sentiments – that empowerment, agency and self-led action are essential ingredients in trauma healing. These clinicians are also imperfect, delightful, messy, normal humans – so don't go putting them on a pedestal because it serves neither you or them for you to put them up there.

More and more clinicians are now acknowledging the power of the individual to create their own trauma healing. I'm including some of their voices here to give you confidence that the self-led approach described in this book is theoretically and clinically sound. It pulls together an empowering body of theories, practices and approaches that are evidence-based and widely used in practice to heal childhood trauma. I hope hearing these clinicians helps you feel held, not just by me, but by my entire field.

The clinicians I spoke to are a diverse bunch that represent a lot of different approaches and modalities. Sat Dharam Kaur is a naturopathic doctor and runs Compassionate Inquiry along with Gabor Maté. Dane Ensley builds bespoke, trauma-informed therapeutic teams around his clients. Dr Ingrid Clayton is a clinical psychologist, specialising in the fawn response. Julia Samuels is a psychotherapist and author, specialising in loss and grief. Sheryl Close uses psychotherapy and SE to treat complex trauma and PTSD. Lou LeBentz uses Eye Movement Desensitisation and Reprocessing (EMDR) to help clients process and release trauma. Dr Brad Reedy runs psychotherapeutic programs that focus on self-knowing and self-acceptance as the vehicles for change and healing. Josh Dickson combines surfing and EMDR in his approach to trauma healing and Calum Morrison creates unique, extraordinary adventures for clients to help create deep change.

They all facilitate trauma healing in wonderfully different ways, but each of them empowers their clients into safe, self-led action to do so.

Reality check

More than anything, I want this book to be useful. Recently, at the end of a session, a client said to me: 'It's a relief that you're writing this book because trauma healing isn't accessible or affordable. Anything you can do to pull people in and give clear, logical guidance on how to get from A to Z is very good thing.'

I couldn't agree more. This book is about empowerment and agency, but it's also about reality. And the reality is, many people cannot afford to see a therapist weekly for years to slowly *unfold* their trauma patterns and process their past. A weekly session with a therapist or psychologist in London ranges from about £60 to £400 an hour. In Sydney you'll pay between about $70 and $350. In New York roughly between $150 and $400. If we split the difference and say you'll pay about £/$200 an hour, for twelve months of weekly therapy, taking out time for the odd holiday and birthdays, it will cost a minimum of £/$10,000.

There's a very real need for high-quality, low-cost ways in to trauma healing. I believe in this empowered, self-led approach because I see first-hand the powerful healing it results in. But I also believe it is morally right to increase accessibility whenever and however we can.

Yes, but . . .

The self-led approach I describe in detail in Part Two of the book is safe and empowering. But no approach is *for everyone*.

If you're extremely dysregulated and get stuck for long periods of time in very intense emotions, if you experience intense flashbacks from the past or if you have a cluster of different psychiatric diagnoses, it's likely that you'll need to work with a trauma-trained therapist or practitioner before you can fully utilise the self-led approach. This is not because a clinician has all the answers. It's not because you need fixing. It's about something much more gentle and lovely than this. It's about *co-regulation* – which is the glorious, astonishing way that our nervous system mirrors the nervous system of the people around us. In childhood this mechanism was problematic because our developing nervous system was mirroring (i.e. copying and learning from) the nervous system of adults who were often dysregulated (e.g. stressed, in survival, shut down, etc). But in trauma healing this mechanism is a super power. As we work with a regulated trauma-trained therapist our nervous system mirrors theirs, and over time we move back into regulation and balance. This co-regulation, then, lays the foundation for the self-led journey.

On page 155 you'll find a lot more information about when and why you may need to work with a clinician. There's more information about this, specific to when to work with an Internal Family Systems (IFS) practitioner, on page 266 too.

If you sense this applies to you and you're feeling dismayed, let me tell you one of the Principles of Self-led Integration: stretch but don't stress. This principle reminds us that to heal we have to learn when to say no, when to walk away and when to reach for support. Working with a practitioner because you are authentically connecting to your reality, feeling that you're at your limit and taking action in response is what this self-led thing is all about.

Even if you're sensing that you may need a little extra scaffolding and co-regulation before you dive into Part Two, Part One of this book is for *everyone*. Read this to get a deeper understanding of childhood trauma and autopilot and come back to the rest when you're ready.

The problem and the solution

This book is divided, very simply, into two parts. Part One is all about The Problem and Part Two is all about The Solution. Part One is deliberately short – I want to create a book that sits in the energy of the solution and of hope, rather than in the energy of the problem.

Part One: The Problem

In Chapter One, I use my own wake-up call to illustrate the problem we face: unconscious autopilot, disconnection and repetition. In Chapter Two, I explain why and how childhood trauma locks us into unconscious survival patterns and disconnects us from our self, our agency, other people and the world. Chapter Three (the final chapter of Part One) is all about the consequences of living in the problem.

Part Two: The Solution

Chapter Four explains the process of trauma healing – there's a lot of theory and detail here, so you understand what you're aiming for and how to get there. Chapter Five explains more about the self-led approach and how it links to integration and neuroplasticity. This chapter also includes The Principles of Self-led Integration. These principles are your handrails, designed to guide you through the self-led journey safely. Chapters Six, Seven, Eight and Nine are in-depth guides to self-led healing. One by one, these chapters will teach you how to learn and integrate the Four Core Capacities of trauma healing:

1. The capacity to signal safety to your nervous system and self-regulate.
2. The capacity to move into presence, observation, curiosity and clarity.
3. The capacity to receive yourself with perspective and compassion, as a wise, loving adult.
4. The capacity to unlock your agency and take self-led action.

In Chapter Six, the first of the in-depth guides, you'll learn how to increase your capacity to self-regulate and feel safer in your body. This includes detailed information on how to harness the power of your imagination to help you feel safe and create change. In Chapter Seven, you'll learn how to increase your capacity for presence, observation and curiosity. Next, in Chapter Eight, you'll learn how to develop your capacity to respond to yourself as a wise, loving adult and undertake deeper self-led trauma-healing work. In Chapter Nine, you'll learn how to unlock your agency and integrate your capacity to take empowered self-led action so you can stop reacting and start creating. Lastly, in Chapter Ten, I add any last little nuggets of wisdom so you're fully armed to create and implement real change in yourself and your life.

Who this book is for

This book is for people who feel disconnected from their own agency and power to create positive change. It's for people who sense they need to heal but don't know how or are scared to do so. It's for people who've recently had their own wake-up call, and people who sense that their mind, body and life are calling them to act now.

It's for those who sense that their own trauma relates to a loss of agency and so intuitively know that to heal they must, in some way, reclaim their power.

It's also for those who are in therapy but feel stuck or disempowered and for those too afraid or resistant to go to therapy. And it's for the millions who cannot afford therapy or have no access to good, trauma-informed, empowering therapeutic support.

It's also for those who simply do not agree that someone else is required to 'fix' you, and for those who do not feel aligned with the current patriarchal model of mental health.

I need to pause for a moment, because I'm aware that although many of the previous descriptions relate to me before the diagnosis, I was oblivious to just how stuck I was. I would have read those descriptions and thought, *Nope, not me.*

So how do people like me, with their head firmly in the sand, find a way to relate to this book?

To address this, I'll add that this book is for anyone who knows or senses they have unresolved trauma and who are simultaneously aware that they've been avoiding this truth. It's for anyone who senses that somewhere deep inside them, something needs healing. Because this sentiment would have resonated with me before I was diagnosed. I knew there was more to heal. Perhaps you do too.

Privilege and uncomfortable irony

After confidently listing 'who this book is for', I want to acknowledge my privilege. I was born into a white body and into the dominant culture. I am middle-class and I went to university. 'My' culture is the one that has colonised and capitalised. 'My' culture came up with the disempowering, predominantly white, middle-class, expert-led mental health system. 'My' culture is highly problematic in this world of trauma healing.

To write meaningfully about disempowerment and loss of agency, I have to acknowledge that my privilege has given me health, wealth, resources and a sense of belonging. I am seen and heard in a way that many others are not. I am systemically empowered in a way that others are not. Just being able to write this book demonstrates the privilege and empowerment I experience, where others do not.

Members of minority groups and marginalised communities experience high levels of financial trauma, racial trauma, systemic trauma and intergenerational trauma. People in these groups and communities are often born into a systemic loss of agency and lack of choice. They often inhabit a body, culture and identity that mainstream culture systemically undermines, neglects or attacks.

The dominant, colonial culture has provided many of the 'empowering, self-led solutions' I offer in this book. I hear the irony and it makes me wince. For this reason, the solutions I present here may feel, and be, unrelatable and inappropriate for some.

I cannot change my privilege, but I can acknowledge it, and the bigger issues we collectively face as we try to empower ourselves and heal trauma.

Part 1

The problem

Chapter One

The wake-up call

Before I share the dark underbelly of my most recent *new lowest point*, I want you to know who I am professionally. Maybe then, as well as teaching you how to heal yourself, this book will also help soften any black-and-white thinking you may have around success and healing. Because I am deeply, profoundly imperfect. I fail at something every day. I cannot multi-task, I'm frequently socially awkward, I'm always learning . . . *and* I have a thriving, purpose-led career. I have helped thousands of people heal and I have healed my own mind and body in a deep and profound way. I believe that the more I show you just how very human and flawed I am, the better. I believe that our connection will be forged through our humanness, not through any perfection you might unconsciously ascribe to me as the author of a book.

This book is an invitation to question the whole idea that someone else knows more about how to heal you than you do. Including me. I can tell you what I know, but ultimately we are just humans coming together to share and heal. I'm aware, as I say this, of the irony that the cover of this book has the words 'trauma expert' under my name in huge letters. If you could put this down to marketing, and to that humanness I just referred to, I'd appreciate it.

My approach

I researched trauma for fifteen years as an academic and I now run a busy private practice working with adults who have unresolved relational trauma from childhood. My entire approach, and everything I do, is designed to empower clients to create meaningful, sustainable change internally and externally (because the change is the healing). I'm a coaching psychologist, not a clinical psychologist, and this is not accidental. Coaching psychologists use psychological concepts, approaches and theories to empower clients to build their own capacity to heal. Because, yes, to heal trauma we need to release and process our pain, but we also need to build resources and resilience. We need more of what has been missing – resilience, flexibility, safety, connection, adult perspective, regulation, confidence, compassion, self-efficacy (that is, self-belief) and agency. Building and integrating what is limited or missing to create change and healing is the foundation of my approach, and this book.

I've also trained in Internal Family Systems (IFS), a leading therapy designed to heal childhood trauma. I chose this modality because not only does it help release and process the pain of childhood trauma, it's inherently empowering. Woven into the foundation of an IFS approach is the central message of this book: that we each have the power to self-heal and as we unlock this power we create a whole new way of being and relating. My practice has taught me that this approach – which is all about empowerment, agency and self-connection – leads to life-changing results for adults with unresolved childhood trauma.

I feel very passionate about the need to increasingly move trauma out of the medical and clinical domain. Trauma is part of the human condition. We've all experienced it and we all have unresolved trauma in our systems. Yes, some have more than others. But the more we collectively know about trauma the clearer it becomes that it's something that applies to every single one of us. My hope is that we'll come to view trauma as we do other universal concepts within psychology – as existing on a *spectrum*. Trauma, like anxiety, self-control or self-esteem, is something we all have. We're all somewhere on the trauma spectrum. Arguably this is the most important spectrum of all because our place on it determines many other aspects of our health, wellbeing and life. Just like anxiety, trauma can be a state that we exist in, and/or it can come and go. Either way, it's inherently human and nothing to be ashamed of. Most importantly, it's very possible to move yourself down to the lower end of the spectrum.

Not only has it become patently clear that trauma is something we all experience, it has also become increasingly clear that trauma no longer sits within a purely psychological/psychotherapeutic domain. Trauma is about the nervous system and the body. It's about our physical health. It's about the way live. It's about our social lives. It's about our families and communities. It's about our thinking. It's about our compulsions and addictions. It's about the way we move and the way we breathe. It's about the way we cope with stress.

It's about our self-concept and identity. It's about how and when we flourish and move into flow. It's about pretty much everything that makes up being a human.

Because of the breadth and complexity of trauma – because it balloons from the nervous system into many facets of our being over time – it has also become clear that each of us needs to take an active role in our healing. One-to-one sessions with a trauma practitioner are important for many of us (myself included). But it's becoming increasingly clear that trauma healing is something that we must each take ownership of. We can create as much, if not more, healing in the hours outside of therapy sessions as we can during the one hour a week we may choose to see a practitioner.

I believe trauma healing is a call to action. It's an active, self-led process that requires different, contrasting daily experiences to the repetition we've been stuck in. We must act, move, change, flow, release and courageously learn to do things differently. But the problem we face is that trauma has us tightly, rigidly stuck in an old way of doing things. On a deep subconscious level parts of us believe changing is not safe, so without even realising it, we fear, resist and avoid change.

Before we carry on, I want to take a moment to acknowledge the unfairness of the problem we face. It's not fair to expect those with childhood trauma to solve a subconscious problem they cannot see or feel. It's not fair that change is so hard won. It's not fair that it often takes a traumatic wake-up call to reveal the problem to us. It's not fair that we face a problem we were handed by someone else. It's not fair, no. As we move forward together I want you to know that I see and feel the injustice on our behalf. I see your pain *and* I know that we can create a different life experience for you, one that's softer and kinder and *fairer* than the one you've been handed.

Crisis and hope

In this moment, I'm writing in my office on a balmy summer's day in England. The sky is a bright, clear blue. Speckled sunshine flows in through the windows and there's a warm, gentle breeze. I can hear the soft coo of a wood pigeon, and further away, the soft hum of someone mowing their lawn. My big Bernese Mountain Dog is lying on the floor next to me snoring loudly. I feel calm, anchored and present.

All is well, I am safe and I am home. And I am profoundly grateful for the simple deliciousness life offers me in this moment.

Seven years ago, a crisis was unfolding in my body and my life. I wish I could rewind time and show myself this future moment – the sun, the peace, the wellness, the gratitude. I wish I could show myself that all would be well, because at times I felt hopeless and beaten down.

If you or someone you love are in the midst of what feels like a life-altering crisis, my dearest hope is that my story will give *you* hope. Because hope matters greatly. I'm not talking about fake, giddy positivity. I'm not talking about gaslighting yourself and pretending your grief, fear or anger doesn't exist.

Life is incredibly hard sometimes and stating this, and being in this hardness and pain, is essential to healing. Life is hard, often. Life feels unfair, often. *And*, within our pain, there can also be a glimmer of something softer and gentler.

I hope this book can be a glimmer for you. I hope that through my honesty you will become willing to believe that healing and change are possible, no matter how bad things seem right now.

Trauma is the outcome of experiences that feel too much for us to cope with – you can read more about this in Chapter Two. For now, and before I tell you about my own too-much-experience, I want to reassure you that no matter how hard life seems right now, it will pass. Perhaps life feels too much for you right now. Perhaps you're having your own wake-up call – whether you've experienced bereavement, a diagnosis, a job loss, a relationship breakdown, illness, addiction, family breakdown, financial crisis or any impactful life event that feels *too much*.

Before we move on I need you to hear me when I say that everything is going to be okay. It might not be precisely the same, but it will be *okay*. One day you're going to feel calm, anchored and present. You're going to feel the gentle breeze and the warmth of the sun on your skin. You're going to feel safe and *home*.

This will pass. All will be well.

After Diagnosis (AD)

The day my neurologist diagnosed me with multiple sclerosis (MS) will forever be imprinted in my memory. I was sitting on my bed anxiously waiting for the phone to ring. I remember struggling to catch my breath – aware of both the terror of impending doom and the anxious, clinging desperation that the worst might not come to pass. Despite mounting evidence that I was unwell, part of me really did think he would say everything was okay. That he'd made a mistake. That I was simply tired and overworked. I felt kicked in the gut when he said, in a weirdly joyful tone of voice, 'The last scan has proved it – you've got MS!'

He seemed really rather pleased that, after months of scans and uncertainty, he was able to join the dots for me. I was . . . less pleased, and started crying. After an appropriate amount of time my neurologist – a lovely bespectacled chap from Oxford with a posh British accent – said, with complete bemusement:

'I'm really quite confused about why you're crying. You'll be absolutely fine. This doesn't mean what you think it means.'

This bizarre exchange continued for some time, with my neurologist giddily explaining how medical understanding and treatment of MS had advanced while I quietly sobbed. After I put the phone down I called my dearest friend.

'I've got MS,' I said, stumbling over words I'd never uttered before.

'Okay,' she said calmly. 'We can deal with that.'

FYI, she was right. We could.

I have a huge smile on my face as I write this because I can see just how lovely, and just how important, this first reponse to *the news* was. So very lovely, and so very important, indeed.

I didn't tell many other people for a long time. My life had tilted on an axis I didn't see coming. I struggled for air. At times I was certain I would die from the grief of losing a future I thought was no longer mine.

I took time off work so I could begin to process and understand what *the news* meant. It's interesting to remember what helped me cope day-to-day. The idea that the diagnosis was a *plot twist* rather than *the end of the story* was profoundly, inexplicably helpful. There was a lightness to the idea that I clung onto. It helped me see a future. It helped me be curious and open. It helped me move into flexibility, and eventually, acceptance.

Due to my own personal plot twist, I've now met a lot of women with MS. All of them have opted for different treatments and approaches to healing. But they share a strength, wisdom and hope that is rare to find. They're also thriving. I know this could sound trite. I know many other people are struggling with chronic illness. But I can only speak to what I've personally witnessed: healing, growth, strength and transformation in direct response to crisis and illness.

Another thing these women have in common is the trigger that directed their immune system to attack them. All of the women I've spoken to cite grief, chronic stress or trauma as the starting point. I should mention that this is true for me too. Eye-wateringly true, in fact.

Like an odd bible parable, my life is now BD (Before Diagnosis) and AD (After Diagnosis). Thirty-six months BD I became highly stressed. Twenty-four months BD I moved from 'highly stressed' to 'only-dogs-can-hear-the-decibel-stressed'. Eighteen months BD my childhood trauma was intensely triggered and I was retraumatised. Fourteen months BD I had the first MS symptom.

In the aftermath of the diagnoses, I was in almost daily contact with a naturopath, Fiona, who specialises in MS because she has it. Witnessing her strength, health and laughter was, I believe, just as powerful as the nutritional advice she provided me. She gave me hope and *this* made all the difference. A beautiful example of why self-led healing isn't about doing it alone.

One month AD, Fiona said, 'You can change your diet, exercise and take all the meds in the world, but unless you learn to deal with your stress it won't make any difference.'

It was extremely painful, humbling and *new* to be viewed in this way – as someone who was stuck, stressed and unwell.

But I knew she was right. I knew that my stress, which was driven by the childhood trauma I still carried, had contributed to the crisis I found myself in.

The months following the diagnosis were a weird old time, as you can imagine. I spoke to Fiona. I met friends for tear-filled lunches. I spoke to the women I've already mentioned, all of whom were friends of friends, rallying to help me come to terms with the news.

Every morning, as soon as I woke up, I drank celery juice. Hilariously, I can't even remember why I leaned on celery as the thing that would stitch back together the holes in my nervous system. Someone said it would help, so I did it. The memory of this terrible, bitter, light-green start to the day makes me want to throw up. I'm palpably relieved I'm no longer in the celery juice phase.

Once the kids had left the house for the day I sat down on the sofa and did what I had wanted to do every minute since I had woken up 90 minutes previously: close my eyes.

This is one of the strongest, most visceral memories from this time – the intense need to close my eyes, to retreat into darkness, to stop the light from entering my eyes and the sound from entering my ears. My body was calling me to help it, telling me what it needed, but life and my old patterning relentlessly called me in the opposite direction.

Closing my eyes brought sensory relief but not *actual* relief. Although it felt so good to block out the world, the small act of closing my eyes didn't stop the rising panic and terror. Often it actually it made it worse.

In her wisdom, Fiona had tasked me with 'doing nothing'. She'd told me that this would be almost impossible to start with, but that I needed to work up to being able to *do nothing* for two minutes.

'How do I do nothing?' I had asked.

'The best way to do nothing is to close your eyes, and simply listen,' she had replied. 'It's a lost art,' she added.

So this is what I did. I closed my eyes and listened to the birds and the wind in the leaves for a few seconds. Then I felt the panic and pressure and overwhelm rising so I had to stop. Now, with hindsight, I can see the power and importance of these few seconds. They were the first step I took towards a different type of existence. They were my first act of connection and self-care in a very, very long time.

I was extremely careful about who I spoke to following the diagnosis – about whose energy, words and attitude I would allow into my space and near my mind and body. Because I, in my gloriously black and white mind, was beginning to believe that I had only two options:

One, I could give up and sink into trauma and illness.

Or, two, I could trust that I would heal and that, although it would be different, everything would be okay.

Looking back, I suppose anyone who knew me understood that I'd choose the second option. But for me, as I grappled with the reality of the diagnosis, option one felt very tempting.

When I made the choice to believe that everything would, somehow, be okay, I once again defined who I am in relation to *a difficult thing*. I stood up and, without actually saying it, told the world who I am. I am hopeful. I am resilient. I am someone who is quite used to the shit hitting the fan and having to figure out how to get back up. I am a psychologist who believes trauma and nervous system dysregulation are the root cause of most mental and physical issues. And, most importantly, I believe the body – driven by the power of the mind and the nervous system – wants to heal and can heal.

Before Diagnosis (BD)

In the two years prior to the diagnosis I was chronically stressed, overworking, adrenalised, disconnected from my body and, although I did my level best to hide it, socially anxious. *Intense* is the most accurate word to describe how I experienced my inner and outer worlds. I was finishing a PhD, which anyone will tell you is a tough time. This, in and of itself, would have led to an intense year. But my subconscious, trauma-led response to 'a tough time' has always been to make it tougher. My first act of making it tougher was to add in having my third child. During a time when I needed rest, when my other two children needed what remained of their mother's already divided attention, I chose to get pregnant. My third child is pure heaven, don't get me wrong. But nonetheless I can see in retrospect that the timing, twelve months before I had to hand in my doctoral thesis, was an *interesting* choice.

It gets better. Two months after my daughter was born, and in the midst of writing up and submitting the thesis, I decided we should emigrate. So now I'm breastfeeding a child, looking after two high-energy children, writing a PhD thesis, packing up a house and obsessively researching houses and schools in Australia.

I sat my viva for the PhD two weeks before we got on the plane. I remember trying to make a joke of it all – smiling in a strained, disconnected way at the chaos and intensity.

I recall a feeling of pressure like nothing I'd ever experienced before and a deep panic. There was a rising sense that

I needed to stop what was happening and abort mission because it was all too much. I felt trapped, not just because we'd set the juggernaut of emigrating in motion, but also by my own need to prove myself and find something *better*.

What I told people, and still tell people, is that we moved to Australia because of Brexit. In part this is true, but I think a more honest answer is that we decided to move to Australia because life suddenly felt terribly hard. Rather than slowing down and attending to the feelings of discomfort, I made life more complicated so I wouldn't have to see or feel these things. Instead of standing still and feeling, I started running faster.

I wasn't conscious of this, but this pattern has existed since I was a child. If it feels painful, go faster, do more. Ignore the painful feelings, ignore the need to rest, ignore the panic. Keep smiling, keep joking, keep doing, keep *performing*. Disconnect from it all and keep going. This subconscious way of coping first developed when I was a small child, in response to a sexual boundary violation that I told no-one about. The experience was too much for me so I moved strongly and intensely into survival.

The 'told no-one' part of my history is highly pertinent. The lack of connection goes a long way to explain why this experience embedded in me the way it did – weaving itself into my mind, body and beliefs about myself and the world. Left to their own devices these experiences cause havoc. This sums up childhood trauma: the emotional disconnection we experience means that during a crisis we go inwards, into reactions, patterns and beliefs that cause us harm, because we feel we have no other choice.

Because I was dysregulated and in survival mode I went on to experience more traumatic reactions. This is how trauma works – one trauma sets up, or primes us, for the next. So, there's more I could tell you – more moments, more trauma, as I moved through childhood into my teens and early adulthood. But I won't. Not because I'm ashamed, not because I don't know, not because I can't, but because I care for you and your nervous system. As you move through this book you'll notice that although I include client case studies, I do not give much detail about their traumatic experiences. I do this because at best it's unnecessary and at worst it's triggering.

To heal, you do not need details of others' pain, but you do need to understand how an experience that is simultaneously terrifying *and* too much for us impacts our mind, body, sense of self and behaviour. This is why I mention one of my own childhood traumas here – to help you join the dots. I hope you can see that the subconscious autopilot we get stuck in as adults often has its roots in a moment long ago that was, somehow, too much for us. So many of us are still running from an old pain. Healing happens when we feel safe enough to stop running so we can gently start to see and feel the things we've been trying to get away from.

When I arrived in Australia I was still running. I was scared and in need of support, but in response I doubled down on self-sufficiency and ran faster. In response to my own fear that I was failing and getting it all wrong, I became harder on myself. In response to my increasing sense of panic, I tried harder to get it all right. In response to the burgeoning sense of shame and disconnection, I moved further away from people. There was only work and stress and worry. Only fear and an automatic response to fear that created more stress. At times I knew I needed to do it differently but my old protective patterning had me trapped like glue, pulling me back into old behaviours, beliefs and ways of being. I was frozen in every sense of the word – too afraid to put a toe out of line, even though I could sense that the path I was on was harming me.

I dearly wish I could tell you a different story – one that involved me slowing down, establishing boundaries and caring for myself as I deserved. But I can't do this. I can only tell you the truth, my truth, about the years I was lost in The Problem.

My re-telling of AD and BD might be an uncomfortable read, perhaps even a triggering read if you've had a similar experience. If you feel wobbly, untethered and unsafe please take a moment to help your body feel a little safer. Then turn back to the page and read the 'Crisis and hope' bit again. Because the most important thing I want to convey is that healing is possible. I am now very much okay. This is the context I want you to anchor into: yes, shit happens, but the mind and body really can heal. Sometimes we even look back and see that the very event that we thought was a catastrophe was actually a springboard into a whole new way of living.

Reality

The MS diagnosis was like having all the denial ripped away at once. A bucket of reality was dumped on my head. I saw the unresolved trauma that had been triggered. I saw that I had been in survival mode, oscillating between fight-flight and freeze BD and between freeze and collapse AD. I saw the stress, the adrenaline and the chronic disconnection from my body. I saw the dangerous contradictions in my life and my recovery. I saw the lack of self-care. I saw the lack of emotional connection. I saw that I was not happy, but had been trying to pretend I was. Mainly, though, the truth I became aware of was that the way I had been living was not working. I realised I needed to do things differently. I'm guessing, given that you're here with me now, you too have a sense that you need to do things differently. I hope you do. I hope there's a growing willingness in you to learn a different way. I hope that my story will help you sense that anything is possible once you're willing to truly change.

I need to add that despite my own sudden, acute awareness of the need for change, change itself was a painfully slow process. This wasn't a triumphant sprint to wellness. My healing was created from micro-changes almost imperceptible to the human eye. I had to take it a day at a time, sometimes an hour at a time. This is how I healed my trauma, my mind, my body and my sense of self, and this is how you'll heal too: by creating small, almost undetectable, changes to how you relate to yourself and the world, and then doing it again tomorrow. Waking up is not enough. We need to wake up and then *act*.

Clients contact me for many reasons. Some are in the middle of a life crisis like a relationship breakdown, a diagnosis or a job loss. Others get in touch for the opposite reasons: despite the white picket fence or the career they've always dreamed of, internally they *feel* in crisis. For these clients, it's the contradiction rather than the crisis that calls them to this work. Of course, it's not black and white. Some clients sit in-between the life crisis and the contradiction: just about functioning, but with a new awareness of the problems in their life as well as in their mind and body.

Whether the crisis is internal or external, or whether it's a little bit of both, the *thing* clients have been pushing down and avoiding has become undeniable and intolerable. For one reason or another, their pain and trauma has pierced its way into conscious awareness, and it hurts.

As a practitioner, I can see and feel the power and potential that exists in these first painful moments of awareness. As a human being who has experienced a great many moments of pain piercing conscious awareness, I know – god, how I know – how terrifying these moments can feel. Acute awareness of a pain, a problem or a truth we've been avoiding, coupled with not enough support, no solution in sight and no understanding of how to find a solution is, of course, horrific.

It's horrific in large part *because* we've spent decades denying and avoiding the pain, problem or truth. Because we've so adeptly pushed away *the painful thing* that stems from our childhood trauma, we have no tools now to face it. We cannot tolerate it. This is what trauma does – it locks us into patterns of avoidance and disconnection so we become increasingly unable to tolerate *reality*.

Outside of conscious awareness our nervous system decided that the painful thing was too much for us to handle and moved us into fight-flight-freeze. Now, as a triggered traumatic reaction unfolds we move into old ways of coping that we first started using in childhood. Without realising it, we're doing all we can to consciously avoid *the painful thing* and the more we avoid it, the less we can tolerate it. So when it does pierce our conscious awareness our whole system screams, 'This is too much for me.'

My clients are all in a painful process of coming into awareness. They are coming out of trauma-led patterns of avoidance and disconnection, and becoming able to see and feel their trauma and their truth. This is a good thing. But is also very shit indeed. I remember describing how gut-wrenchingly, existentially awful I felt thanks to this new awareness, to my own psychotherapist. This lovely therapist, Yvette, said:

'You're in the most painful, but most powerful place. It's called *conscious incompetence*. The fog is clearing and you're becoming aware but you don't yet have any tools to do things differently. You can see it but can't yet change it.'

Conscious incompetence – what a terrifying but excellent concept. To heal we must move from unconscious incompetence (totally unaware, automatically repeating trauma-led patterns) to conscious incompetence (painfully aware of the repetition and patterns), so we can then become consciously competent (able to slow down, make different choices and respond differently) and eventually move into unconscious competence (automatically making different choices without having to try so hard).

Trauma practitioners are trained to very slowly move clients out of denial and autopilot and into reality. This describes a lot of the work I do with clients in my own practice. I do this very slowly and very respectfully. If there's too much 'reality' at once my clients are triggered and the work has to stop.

Reality is what we're aiming for, always. I want you to be able to stand in your own reality, your own truth and your own life. I want you to be able to see your own trauma-led patterns without moving into avoidance, panic or shame. I want you to be able to hold your head up high and remain anchored in your adult self as you walk through adulthood, neither minimising or catastrophising what is real for you. The more 'in reality' you can be (awake, connected to your body and emotions, present, aware), the less 'in trauma' you are. And the less 'in trauma' you are, the greater your power and potential to make a different choice. Oddly, then, coming into our reality actually enables us to change it.

I don't want this

Sat Dharam Kaur is a naturopathic doctor and yoga teacher and works alongside renowned trauma specialist and physician Gabor Maté. Together they created Compassionate Inquiry – a new compassion-led approach to healing childhood trauma. Sat Dharam kindly agreed to be interviewed for this book, and I'd like to share her response to the very first question I asked her: 'Why do so many of us need a rock bottom to snap us into conscious awareness?' Here's what she said:

When we hit rock bottom our defences break apart, which is a very good thing. Then we have to reassemble ourselves back together, hopefully a little bit differently than we were assembled before, recognising that we don't need to do or be all the things we thought we needed to do or be either to please other people or to perform for other people or live up to other people's expectations.

It's that ripping apart of the personality that sometimes addiction does, sometimes an illness does, an accident or a life crisis does. But in each case, these are important transition points in our lives to become the new version of ourselves. Hopefully a more authentic version of ourselves.

It doesn't have to be rock bottom, though. Sometimes there's just a recognition that there's something missing. There may be a sense of lack of purpose, lack of joy, lack of meaning. There'll be this emptiness if we're not living in connection with our true self or connected with our body and emotions.

Whatever we get, whether it's an accident or an illness or emptiness, there's a teaching in it. It's our spiritual teacher. So the addiction can be our spiritual teacher. The chronic illness can be our spiritual teacher. Everything is like our spiritual teacher if we allow it. But we have to look at it and ask ourselves: How can I learn from this? Not because I did anything wrong, but because there's something I'm meant to see that I've not been seeing – part of me I'm meant to retrieve that I haven't retrieved yet. What is available to me when I fully give myself to this process that's asking me to look at something?

There's this quote by [the writer and spiritual teacher] Almaas that Gabor quotes: 'The problematic situations in your life are not chance or haphazard . . . They are specifically yours, designed specifically for you by a part of you that loves you more than anything else. The part of you that loves you more than anything else has created roadblocks to lead you to yourself. That part of you loves you so much that it doesn't want you to lose the chance. It will go to extreme measures to wake you up.'

It's not the universe doing it. It is ourselves wanting to be whole: conjuring up this magic trick to make it happen for us. As we face the pain and the problem we still say 'I don't want this' – that's part of it. It's a process. And 10 years or 20 years or 30 years or 40 years later, we'll get it – we'll understand it.

I do not know what's going on in your life as you read this. Perhaps you're in the middle of a life crisis or perhaps you're becoming aware of a contradiction between what you present to the world and how you really feel. What I want for you, and what Sat Dharam and Gabor Maté are calling you to, is authenticity and awareness. But conscious awareness isn't the same as lying down and accepting our fate. Moving out of trauma-led autopilot and into reality is about becoming present, but it's also about reclaiming our free will, agency and choice. We *look* so we can learn. Then as we say 'I don't want this' we create something different for ourselves.

Chapter Two

The why

This chapter is designed to help you understand why we end up on autopilot but are unaware of it. I need to explain *the why* because a) it makes me seem less mad BD and b) I hope it will increase your clarity and compassion about why you might have struggled to take action and implement real change before now.

The short answer to *why?* is: childhood trauma (i.e. developmental, relational and/or complex trauma from childhood) and the subconscious nervous system-led patterns it locks us into. Trauma is like glue. It's insidious, sneaky and weirdly intoxicating. The fear, the anxiety and worry, the avoidance, the chronic stress, the overworking, the pushing people away, the people-pleasing, the hiding and every other survival adaptation we've leaned on feel like the solutions we need. They call to us, urging us to rely on them and trust them. They have us all fooled because what they promise is safety, but what they give us is an unsettling sense that we are not safe at all. Our trauma-led ways of coping create the problem they're physiologically designed to solve, and they do it in such a slippery way that even those committed to trauma healing can struggle to see and feel just how stuck they are.

To change, we first have to be able to see the reality of ourselves and our lives, and this is pretty hard given that we're trying to see something that doesn't want to be seen. This chapter is designed to help you see things a little more clearly because before we can move into The Solution, we have to get clear on The Problem we face.

Yadda yadda

When I wrote my first book, trauma was still a big, scary, misunderstood thing, so my explanation of it felt fresh and useful. Trauma is now a widely used term. I love that we're all increasingly comfortable having a conversation about it, *and* it puts me in a bit of a weird position as I write my second book. I don't want to bore you ('dear god please don't let them be bored', thought every author). But I do need to explain trauma well enough to inform and empower you. I've also come to realise that although there's a lot of trauma noise out there, not all of it is helpful or correct. So although this chapter might seem to cover familiar ground – although it may all feel a bit 'yadda yadda trauma yadda yadda', please, you know, do actually read it.

Trauma is weird

Traumatic reactions are weird. They're simultaneously specific mechanisms that activate during a scary experience *and* a broad range of responses your mind and body deploy to ensure the scary experience doesn't happen again. As I explain how a physiological mechanism our bodies have evolved to protect us leads to a life lived in survival and disconnection, I hope you'll also get clearer on your own trauma and the patterns it's trapped you in.

Before I get into the weeds, and for anyone who appreciates brevity, I'm going to give you a comprehensive (read as *irritatingly academic*) definition of trauma. Although overarching definitions are deeply satisfying to write, they also tend to be inaccessible to most people. I'm including this explanation here to create structure, but I'm also going to spend the rest of this chapter, and the next, unpicking and explaining what all this means in real human terms.

Trauma: An irritatingly academic but satisfying definition

Trauma is an incomplete nervous system survival reaction to a perceived threat that feels too much for us to handle or comprehend. The intense survival response (fight, flight, freeze, fawn and collapse) floods our mind and body with arousal hormones (e.g. adrenaline and cortisol). We experience this as different physiological symptoms, such as anxiety-like symptoms, dissociation or shut-down; emotions (often fear, terror, anger and shame) and, over time, traumatic beliefs about ourselves, other people and the world such as 'people can't be trusted', 'I'm bad', 'I'm disgusting', 'I'm getting it wrong', or 'The world is unsafe.'

The intense survival response interferes with our cognitive processing, so the threat experience is not processed completely into our long-term memory. Instead the 'memory' exists as an 'unprocessed imprint' (meaning we haven't made sense of it). The experience is stored as sensory information like smells and sounds, physiological information like tension, contraction, physical pain or emotions, or cognitive information like thoughts and beliefs. When our nervous system picks up on reminders of the imprint later in life (such as a certain smell combined with tension in the body) it will move us into the nervous system survival response to try and protect us from what it interprets as another, similar, threat.

To cope with the easily triggered unprocessed trauma and the incomplete survival response that we're trapped in, we develop protective survival adaptations. Over-striving, people-pleasing, compulsive behaviours (like worrying, overeating, undereating, overworking, drinking), isolation and avoidance are all common ways of coping with unresolved childhood trauma. These adaptations reflect what's happening in our nervous system. A clear example of this is how the nervous system's fawn response drives people-pleasing behaviour (see page 55 for more on this).

Every aspect of the survival response is designed to protect us by keeping us away from possible threat and the memory of the threat. From the initial dissociation (e.g. feeling light-headed, spacey and disconnected) to the avoidance strategies we rely on decades later, the traumatic reaction is a process of unconscious avoidance and disconnection designed to keep us safe. But as we unconsciously try to disconnect from the painful emotions, from the imprint of the trauma and from possible threats, we also lose connection to our body, sense of self, safety, other people and the world.

This complex nervous system reaction and the process of unconscious avoidance and disconnection it traps us in is why we get stuck in autopilot. As adults we have a triggered reaction to a threat that we may no longer recall, or that we might never have been able to recall, and our body goes into survival mode. Helping you to understand your deeply ingrained response patterns, and change them, is the goal of this book.

An incomplete response

Perceived threat

Perceived threats to our attachment relationships and core relational connections, to our life and body, or to our resources and security, will trigger our survival response. Anything, then, that threatens our sense of safety will trigger the nervous system's survival response. For a fuller explanation of experiences that commonly feel overwhelmingly threatening, please head to page 6 in the introduction.

If we can't respond to and deal with the threat we move into a traumatic reaction. Given that children are naturally less able to defend themselves or 'deal with' a problem, traumatic reactions in childhood are common. Likewise, whether in childhood or adulthood, when the sense of threat outweighs our internal resources (such as our sense of safety or self-belief) and/or our external resources (for example, support and connection), we move into a traumatic reaction. This is why support matters so much. Traumatic experiences become traumatic because we unconsciously sense that there's no-one standing by us to co-regulate us and help us understand our experience.

No matter what the threat is, the nervous system follows the same response pattern. First it floods us with energy to help us fight or flee by activating the sympathetic nervous system (which functions like a gas pedal in a car, providing us with bursts of arousal energy). If we can't fight or flee, our nervous system moves us into freeze, then swiftly into fawn and then collapse if the threat hasn't resolved. Before we look at the full response, I'll take a moment to explain the initial burst of energy: fight and flight.

Fight-flight: Both feet on the accelerator

Our mind and body are flooded with the arousal hormones cortisol and adrenaline, which give us energy to help us respond to the threat. We commonly experience this flood of hormones as feeling tense and guarded, energised and hypervigilant. Our hearts race and our breathing becomes shallow. Emotionally we might feel edgy, anxious, afraid, irritable or angry.* The sense of threat and all those stress hormones also affect how we think, what we think/say to ourselves and others and the conclusions we come to. We often overthink, obsess, ruminate, plan, panic, worry, hate (self or others), rage, control, judge or blame (self or others).

Freeze: One foot on the accelerator and one on the brake

If we can't respond to and use the sympathetic arousal energy coursing through our body – if we can't run, fight or resolve the situation – and the nervous system senses that we're flooded by too many arousal hormones, it slams on the dorsal vagal brake, the branch of the vagus nerve that slows everything down and moves us into freeze.

Freeze is an odd in-between state where we feel simultaneously adrenalised and on edge *and* are unable to act/move/do because the body is starting to contract. We most commonly

---

* In non-threat situations fight-flight arousal energy can lead to us feeling powerful, motivated and in control.

experience freeze as feeling tense, adrenalised, anxious or edgy, just as in the fight-flight state I described above, while simultaneously feeling on autopilot, floaty and disconnected, stuck, overwhelmed, paralysed or unable to act. Emotionally we can also feel ashamed. Cognitively we feel torn, unable to make a decision, stuck in a loop, flooded, obsessive or confused.

The term *functional freeze* is helpful for many, as it highlights that although we feel disconnected, we've learned to operate in autopilot and push ourselves to carry on from this frozen state.

Fawn: Focused on appeasing another person

We most commonly experience fawn as feeling dissociated and disconnected from our body and sense of self, coupled with an urgent need to submit and pander to another person to ensure we remain safe. Emotionally we tend to feel fixated, anxious and/or ashamed *until* we receive reassurance from the other person. Cognitively we tend to obsess and ruminate on the perceived relational threat and/or about how to repair it. We focus fully on other people and in the process abandon ourselves even more.

Collapse: Both feet on the brake

If the threat continues to feel too big the dorsal vagal brake moves us into complete shut-down. We most commonly experience collapse as feeling as if we're shutting down physically, emotionally and mentally. We have no energy and feel unable to speak, think or move. We often feel dissociated and disconnected from our bodies and the environment. Emotionally we feel 'flat', depressed, despairing, powerless or helpless. Cognitively we struggle to think and have little motivation. We also experience negative or catastrophic thinking and at times obsess, ruminate, worry, hate (self or others) or blame (self or others). The downward momentum of collapse is very different to the activating arousal energy of fight-flight. The body is trying to conserve energy, but even in collapse we still have adrenaline spikes as we panic and try to prevent ourselves from completely sinking.

An ongoing threat

The survival response I've just described is designed to *complete*. The system is meant to flexibly move us into survival and then out of survival once the threat has passed. It is possible, and common, for humans to move into fight, flight or freeze and then through the reaction. The body mobilises and uses the energy and simultaneously senses that the signs of threat have gone and been replaced with signs of safety, such as support, care, connection and calm. It has done its job. We have moved through the response in a flexible way because our nervous system knows we have re-anchored back into safety.

This is not the case for those with *unresolved* trauma. As this term implies, our nervous system response is unresolved. We haven't experienced the divine release and resolution that comes with returning to safety. We live on high alert, oscillating between fight-flight, freeze, fawn and collapse.

Trauma is an *incomplete* nervous system survival response – the nervous system gets stuck in the escalating survival response because it doesn't receive adequate signs that the threat has passed. We are, quite literally, stuck in survival and on autopilot. This need for resolution and signs of safety gives us a clue about how to heal trauma – to heal, the nervous system needs to sense that the threat is over and that you're now safe.

Dysregulation and regulation

The term *nervous system dysregulation* refers to a nervous system that is unable to respond flexibly to stressors and move easily between the parasympathetic (rest) and the sympathetic (arousal) branches. Dysregulation is part of being human – everyone gets stuck and struggles to move up or down from time to time. But for those with unresolved trauma, nervous system dysregulation is the only state we know. Our nervous system reacts quickly and strongly to life's stressors and perceived threats, moving us into sympathetic arousal in an intense way. It resists moving us out of this state because it's become hardwired to keep us alert – it believes we benefit from being kept hypervigilant and on edge.

A regulated nervous system is flexible and responsive. It can mobilise arousal energy via the sympathetic branch when we need to act, move, do and respond. It can also move back into rest and repair via the parasympathetic branch when the need to act has passed. This flexible responsiveness leads to a nervous system that's in flow and has a gentle rhythm – moving up and down like a wave throughout the day.

Those with unresolved trauma have little sense of what regulation feels like in our bodies. We've had little experience of the feeling of expansion and safety that comes as we reconnect back into our body and the present moment. We may have an intellectual sense of what this word 'regulated' means, but we do not know it intimately, with a whole-body awareness.

Trauma healing is synonymous with learning to become regulated. Very slowly, through daily action, we learn to create flexibility, rhythm and flow within our nervous system, and therefore, in our body, mind and life.

Up and down

The nervous system responses I've described above (fight-flight, freeze, fawn and collapse) aren't clearly delineated, either-or categories. We move up and down, reflecting what's going on in the two branches of our autonomic nervous system (ANS), and therefore often straddle different survival states. For example, we can be in freeze, moving up towards fight-flight or, say, fawn, moving down towards collapse. When we describe the survival response, we're trying to name something that's moving – the flood of arousal hormones and energy around the body, controlled by the sympathetic and para-sympathetic branches of the nervous system. These survival responses are states we can live in, but they are the outcome of moving energy/hormones and they can co-exist. We can be in a state of collapse and also be aware of some fight energy, say. I suggest being curious and staying flexible when thinking about your common patterns.

A neural survival map

From the moment you were born your nervous system has been creating a neural survival map based on your experiences and interactions. It has been remembering anything and everything that posed a possible threat to you and harmed you. It paid special attention to *perceived threats that felt too much for you to handle or comprehend* – that is, traumatic experiences. It remembers the threat (such as abandonment, emotional disconnection, conflict, a speeding car, making a mistake, etc.), the harm the threat caused (physical/emotional pain, the conclusions you came to about yourself, and so on) and the corresponding survival response – fight, flight, freeze, fawn and/or collapse. It may be reassuring to know that it remembers good, safe, empowering experiences too.

If your childhood contained many harmful experiences, such as financial instability, chronic stress, an unwell parent, a bullying sibling, emotionally absent, neglectful or abusive parents, a highly critical or shaming parent, a physically abusive parent, an emotionally enmeshed parent, an abusive adult outside of the home and so on, your little nervous system will have organised itself to protect you. It has wired you to survive and as a result you will have spent long periods of time in survival mode as a child and adolescent. You will have been moving between fight-flight (tense and on edge), freeze (overwhelmed and disconnected), fawn (desperately trying to appease and pander) and collapse (lethargy and shutdown).

Your nervous system was creating a survival map for you – minute by minute it was asking itself: who is safe, who is not safe?; when are they safe, when are they not safe?; when am I safe, when am I not safe? This internal survival map becomes more deeply ingrained every time the same threat response is activated. Through use and repetition, your nerve cells (neurons) communicate with each other in a habitual pattern, creating what's known as *neural pathways*. They become stronger, faster and more automatic the more they are used, moving you into freeze, for example, when you feel criticised or shamed. These pathways, used often enough, form a *neural map* that helps you survive.

You still carry your neural survival map. Outside of your conscious awareness it's still there, reading the room, trying to determine: am I safe or am I unsafe? At the smallest indication of a familiar potential threat, such as a tone of voice, a look, a smell, a situation, these neural pathways fire up. Once again, you're flooded and pulled into the same protective response pattern that was laid down all those years ago. You're thrown back into an old reaction – old sensations, emotions, thoughts, beliefs and behaviours. In many ways we become the age we were during the initial trauma – a younger *part* is activated and takes the driver's seat. It's why you can react with such ferocity, why you're suddenly flooded by shame or anger, why you shrink and hide, why you avoid and why you feel you must prove yourself.

This is the autopilot I've been talking about. *This* is why I spent two years in a fog of stress, anxiety and compulsive, fear-driven overworking. *This* is trauma.

Your survival map is designed to ensure you repeat protective behaviours and survival adaptations. It does this to try and keep you safe, but in doing so prevents you from doing the one thing you need to do to heal and grow and thrive: wake up and slowly do things differently. These automatic responses are designed to keep you safe, and let's be honest, they *did* keep you safe. They allowed you to function in the midst of ongoing emotional dysfunction and cope with challenging situations and continue to live. Your map did its job.

We can know that it's time to move out of autopilot *and* we can come to appreciate how hard our nervous system has been trying to keep us safe.

From autopilot to awareness

To give you an example of trauma as an incomplete survival response and a neural map, let me tell you about my client Sophia.

Sophia works for an international agency in Capitol Hill,

Washington DC. She's worked very hard professionally, starting out in different aid agencies and working her way to the top. She is strikingly driven and capable.

Sophia contacted me because of her anxiety, which had skyrocketed over the previous year. She was also experiencing extreme fatigue and having trouble concentrating because of it. For Sophia, given how much her career meant to her, her body's impact on her capacity to work was unbearable. These initial signs of burnout were the 'wake-up call' I've talked so much about. For Sophia, *this* was her red line. Her body's pain, and her trauma, were grabbing her attention and calling her to action.

Sophia no longer had any superiors at the organisation, but she had other partners and executive officers that she had to navigate. One of her colleagues quickly came up in our sessions together as Sophia found him so hard to work with. Roughly speaking, here's how it would go down most days.

During a discussion Sophia's colleague, Nick, would roll his eyes or appear dismissive and irritated. If this happened publicly, in front of other colleagues, Sophia would feel anxious, spaced-out, embarrassed and ashamed. If it happened privately, Sophia would feel intense rage and say something cutting to hurt and demean Nick in return.

This dance had been going on for about nine months, with little change. There was a different dance going on too, though – a dance between Sophia's awareness and avoidance of the issue. Sophia was slowly becoming able to see and feel her automatic reaction.

Sophia's childhood wasn't easy. Her mother died when she was seven years old and she had an extremely tumultuous relationship with her father. He was highly critical and controlling. Sophia recalls her father repeatedly telling her, 'You're useless' when she made a mistake as a child. Now that she is an adult, Sophia's father still frequently calls her useless but couches it as a 'joke'.

From the outside looking in, trauma patterns often appear blindingly obvious. But when we're in them, they're far from clear. Sophia was genuinely surprised when I suggested that the interaction with her colleague was triggering her old survival response because it so closely echoed her childhood experiences with her father. Whether it was her colleague's eye-rolling, his irritability or his dismissive tone, Sophia's nervous system recognised the imprint of her trauma. Outside of her conscious awareness, her neural map catapulted Sophia into her old childhood reaction – freeze and collapse if it was public humiliation, and rage if it happened in private, reminding her nervous system of the confines of her childhood home.

Sophia wasn't ready for more awareness around this. My suggestion went unacknowledged and she changed the subject. That's okay – great, actually – because the client, not the clinician, must lead the pace and direction of change.

Two months later, out of the blue at the start of a session, Sophia said to me: 'Do you know what I realised this weekend, Nick really reminds me of my dad . . .'

Awareness of our triggers (the things that remind us of our trauma and the imprint and wounding it's left us with) and our triggered reactions (the survival adaptation that jumps out of us) isn't the whole picture. There's work to be done once we can see and feel the autopilot and the repetition. But awareness, as always, is the start.

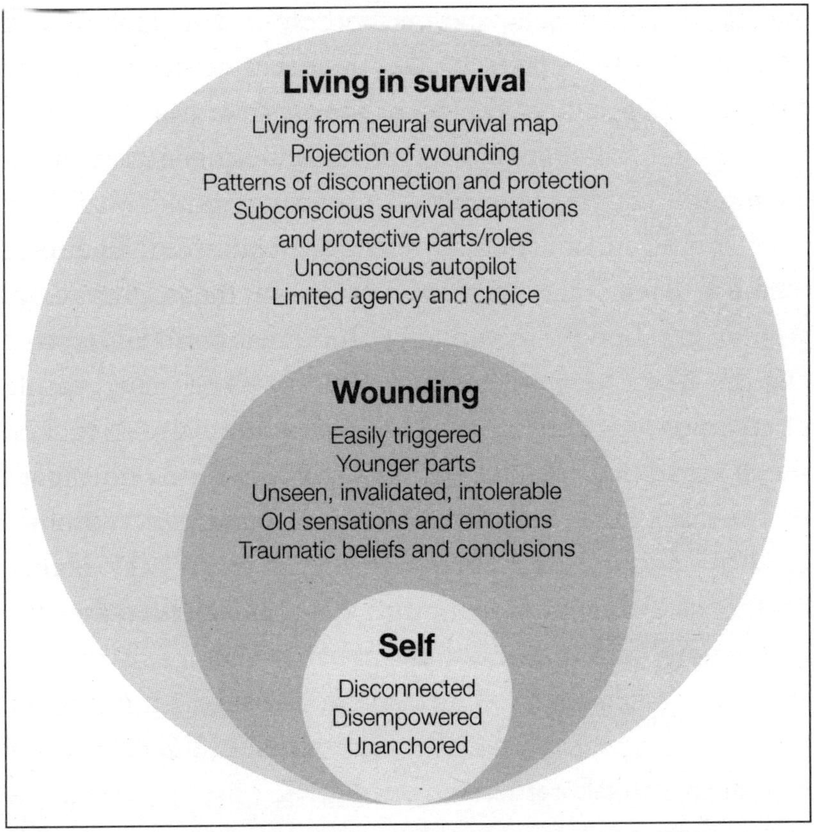

Living in survival

Living from neural survival map
Projection of wounding
Patterns of disconnection and protection
Subconscious survival adaptations
and protective parts/roles
Unconscious autopilot
Limited agency and choice

Wounding

Easily triggered
Younger parts
Unseen, invalidated, intolerable
Old sensations and emotions
Traumatic beliefs and conclusions

Self

Disconnected
Disempowered
Unanchored

Diagram 1: Childhood trauma: The wounding and a life in survival mode

The wounding is the imprint of our traumatic experiences on our bodies, minds and belief systems. It's both the imprint of the threat and the distress it causes. When our nervous system is reminded of this wounding it automatically moves us into hardwired survival adaptations. These disconnect us from our true self in the present moment.

The wounding

The word 'trauma' comes from the Greek for 'wound', and at the most fundamental level, trauma healing is about safely becoming aware of, and safely feeling, our wounding. Over time, we become aware of the 'wound' that traumatic moments, situations, experiences and relationships have created. The wounding is the centre of the trauma. It's the imprint of the initial experience: the mind-body memory of the threat. It's helpful to call it an imprint, not a memory, because trauma 'memories' are very different to normal memories that have been processed, understood and slotted into our long-term memory bank. The imprint consists of the unprocessed, painful mind-body 'memory' of the threat and the harm it caused. When we're triggered in adult life it's because, outside of conscious awareness, our neural survival map has picked up on something related to the wounding and instantly moves us into autopilot – we're thrown into an old survival response.

Our wounding is unique to each of us. It's the bodily, emotional and cognitive imprint of old experiences that felt threatening, and somehow, too much for us. This imprint exists as:

- Disconnected/unprocessed memories, physical sensations and emotions related to the experience.
- Harmful traumatic beliefs and conclusions we formed about ourselves, the world and other people during or immediately after the experience.
- An unmet need, such as the need for connection, safety, love, compassion, validation or acknowledgement.

Later in the book, we'll come to understand this wounding as belonging to younger parts of us that are stuck at the time of the initial trauma. Conceptualising the imprint in this way – as a younger part of us – is extraordinarily helpful and therapeutic. See page 231 for more information on understanding wounding as parts. Until we can see and feel our wounding we project it onto current situations in adult life. It controls us because we aren't aware of it. I'm going to talk more about this in Chapter Three, but I want you to be aware that although your wounding is active and easily triggered, it's buried. Sometimes we get a glimpse of it during a sharp emotional pain, memory or knowing, or when we're flooded with old, intense emotions. Our wounding wants us to see it and heal it, but when we do get this glimpse into our trauma, our survival response kicks in to protect us by disconnecting us from it, because it thinks the trauma is too painful for us to see and feel.

This is what was happening to me in those two years before the diagnosis. Outside of my conscious awareness, my unprocessed wounding had been activated. In response to triggering life experiences that reminded me of my childhood, my wounding increasingly warned me: 'You're unsafe', and 'You're worthless.' In response, and to save me from the pain of these old beliefs, my neural survival map kicked in and moved me into familiar, old ways of coping. These ways of coping felt safe; they felt as if they were the only solution. The solution I knew from childhood was rumination and worry, over-striving, panic, self-abandonment, self-hatred, self-blame, chronic stress and tension. This is what I had done when these beliefs formed in childhood, so as an adult I just followed the same playbook.

I was not unsafe and I was not worthless, but I *projected* this old trauma wounding from my childhood onto my adult life. And as I did, I became trapped in old survival adaptations that created more and more and more and more fear, disconnection and tension, not less.

We come to know our wounding as we become able to move through life with more embodied safety (that is, when our body feels safe, comfortable and calm), conscious awareness, curiosity and compassion. As our nervous system settles, as we begin to reconnect and feel incrementally safer, as we become able to notice and *be with* more emotion and sensation, as we increasingly anchor into our true self and develop self-compassion, we become able to see, feel and 'hold' our wounding.

I hope, as I explain this process, you get a sense of why we all avoid this. The solution you're looking for requires you to see and feel aspects of your past and yourself that are deeply painful. It's okay that you've been avoiding it. It's okay to feel hesitant and resistant to looking at it now.

The ways we survive

To cope with, avoid or manage our wounding we develop different protective strategies and adaptations. These adaptations are designed to keep us safe by keeping us away from the painful memories, sensations, emotions and beliefs at our centre. These adaptations are part of the fight-flight, freeze, fawn and/or collapse response. These adaptations *are* the unconscious autopilot I've talked so much about.

Some of the adaptations, such as hypervigilance, rage or dissociation, are part of the initial flood of hormones, whereas other adaptations, like compulsive busyness, say, come later and over time as the system is wired into survival. I like the term 'survival adaptation', as it makes it clear that we're reacting and adapting to something intensely challenging – the trauma – but you'll notice that I'm not introducing anything new here. The survival response I describe above (pages 53–6) is comprised of two things – the initial wounding and the survival adaptations that the wounding pushes us into.

Some survival adaptations are experienced primarily in the body, such as dissociation, panic attacks, chronic anxiety, tiredness and lethargy. Some are primarily experienced in the mind, like minimising, ruminating, over-planning, hypervigilance, pessimism, catastrophic thinking and so on. Some of these, like excessive self-reliance, isolation, over-working, drinking alcohol, avoiding people and places, compulsive eating, perfectionism and needing to be in control, are behavioural strategies.

Survival adaptations are diverse and unique, which makes it hard to give you an overview. Anything that you consciously or unconsciously do or don't do to manage or avoid your wounding is where they're at. The most important thing for you to know is that the survival adaptations are all designed to protect you from something that links to your wounding. For example:

- A need to control might be trying to protect you from feeling out of control.
- Overthinking, worry and rumination might be trying to help you swerve potential (imagined) future threats.
- Hypervigilance might be trying to protect you from making a mistake.
- A drinking or drug habit might be trying to protect you from feeling uncomfortable emotions that link to your wounding.
- Obsessive tidying might be trying to protect you from feeling bad, worthless or unsafe.
- Pessimism might be trying to protect you from feeling rejected.
- People-pleasing might be trying to protect you from feeling abandoned.

- Avoiding physical touch might be trying to protect you from feeling shame.
- Undereating might be protecting you from feelings of self-disgust, whereas overeating might be helping you get the sense of comfort and connection you crave.
- Overworking or compulsive busyness could be protecting you from feelings of not-enoughness and lack of worth.

Your survival adaptations are protective, not pathological. They're trying to help you and keep you safe. They're the ways we learned to cope with experiences that felt too much for us. There's a logic to all your survival adaptations. They make sense.

For many, it's hard to even begin to consider that a core part of their being might actually be a survival adaptation rather than an adult choice. We want free will, agency and choice, so the idea that some of our ways of being are survival adaptations is extremely confronting.

It's also necessary to consider this idea. How I wish I'd been ready and willing to confront this uncomfortable idea BD. How differently things might have gone if I'd slowed down enough to see and feel that the overworking, the obsessive planning, the hypervigilance, the striving, the emigrating, all of it, was trying to protect me from the unresolved trauma wounding that still existed in my nervous system and my psyche.

Every aspect of the nervous system's survival response is designed to disconnect us to protect us. No matter what type of reaction we're experiencing, it's helpful to consider how it operates to disconnect us from:

- The present moment
- Our body

- Our emotions
- Our adult self
- Other people
- The world
- Spirituality, trust and flow.

As the body contracts and moves into fight-flight-freeze, our thinking and behaviour follow suit, aiming to disconnect us to protect us. It's worth taking a moment to consider what your own survival adaptations disconnect you from. Whether it's hypervigilance, anxiety, compulsive busyness, worry, fear, self-hatred, people-pleasing, dissociation or overwhelm, consider how these things disconnect you from yourself and the world. This disconnection is designed to keep you safe by managing or avoiding emotional pain, discomfort and possible threats, but over time it has precisely the opposite effect, because most of the things we disconnect from are the anchors we need to feel safe, well and whole. Take another look at the list above. These are all basic facets of being, living and relating that every human needs to feel safe. They're the things we need in ourselves and our lives to navigate life, and to grow and thrive.

Trauma healing is, quite literally, a beautiful process of reconnection. We reconnect with our body, our true feelings, the present moment, our adult self, other people and the beauty of the world.

Information overload

Before we move on I want to acknowledge that this is a lot of information. Information overload can be triggering for those with childhood trauma. It can feel too much for us and can trigger our old wounding, activating beliefs like: 'I'm getting it wrong', 'I'm useless', 'I'm a failure', 'I'm in trouble' and so on.

If you're feeling overwhelmed and flooded please remember: You're triggered. You have not done anything wrong. You are safe. This chapter has a lot of information. You do not have to know everything to heal. You don't have to figure it all out. Self-led healing is a journey. We take it one day at a time, sometimes one moment at a time.

I know it's painful not to know and I know it feels profoundly unsafe not to have it all figured out, but it's okay. Can you let this chapter wash over you? Can you try and trust that you heard what you needed to hear? Can you trust that this is an experiential journey, not an intellectual one? You do not have to be an expert, you just need to show up . . . which you have.

Chapter Three

The consequences

We've looked at why we end up stuck in unconscious auto-pilot, repeating behaviours that harm us and unable to change; now we're going to look at the consequences of living life asleep, repeating and on autopilot. *The why* is, of course, childhood trauma – the easily activated wounding and the cascade of survival adaptations that follow. To add some colour to all this 'yadda yadda trauma yadda yadda', I'm going to tell you about the extraordinary women and men I work with on a daily basis, although including them in this section seems a little unfair, really. Like me, the consequences they faced provided their springboard for deep healing, which I'll talk about in Part Two: The Solution. There you'll learn *how* they've created such phenomenal self-led change and healing. But for now, we need to stay in The Problem for just a little while longer.

At a top level, the consequence is that our trauma – the wounding and the multitude of adaptations we've developed

71

to cope with the wounding – directs our life. We build our life on it and around it. This overarching idea is perhaps more important than a list of specific outcomes because the outcomes are so very broad and far-reaching. Our wounding, and the survival adaptations we develop to cope, can take us anywhere. For this reason, someone with unresolved trauma is as likely to be signed off work and unable to leave the house because of chronic anxiety as they are to be travelling from New York to London weekly as CEO of their company. They're as likely to avoid social situations completely as they are to always say 'yes' to any and every invitation. They're as likely to be unassertive and compliant as they are to be aggressive and defiant.

These extremes can only be explained through a trauma framework, and the idea that trauma leads to a life spent either reacting *from* or *to* the wounding. If we react *from* the wounding, we subconsciously design a life that mirrors it. If our wounding tells us we're disgusting, say, we operate from this belief. We might avoid physical touch, rarely buy ourselves new clothes and hide away. We move into our wounding and operate *from it*. Whereas if we react *to* our wounding we subconsciously design a life that buries, avoids and denies it. So if it tells us we're disgusting we construct a life to prove it wrong – perhaps becoming highly flirtatious, obsessed with looking perfect, spending vast amounts on new clothes and needing attention. We move into a performance as a reaction *to* the wounding.

I cannot possibly list all the consequences of living with unresolved childhood trauma. Anything extreme needs to be looked at. More than anything, this word – extreme – is the most helpful guide as you contemplate your own survival adaptations. No matter the direction they take us, the consequences of childhood trauma always look and feel *extreme*.

Contradictions and extremes

My clients are extremely capable humans. They're smart, switched on, loving, conscientious, kind and capable. Many of them also shoulder big responsibilities. They work for international organisations, they're surgeons, they're in charge of emergency departments, they're raising children, they're solicitors, they're app developers, they're CEOs, they're academics, they're renovating houses, they're teachers, they're in the police force, they're documentary makers. I could go on because my client list comprises incredible people who have a lot to give and go the extra mile day in, day out. According to many definitions of success, (you know the ones – the lists of standards we adhere to as proud members of the patriarchal capitalist societies we live in) these people are thriving.

And yet, together in sessions they're acknowledging that they are stuck, stressed, disconnected and frightened. Acknowledging that they carry unresolved relational trauma from childhood. Acknowledging that although the outside often looks sparkly, the inside feels far from it.

My clients are linked through their capability and achievements. They're also linked by their childhood trauma and nervous system dysregulation. This book is largely about this seemingly contradictory fact.

I need to add that many of my clients will not be able to relate to what I'm saying. They will presume I'm referring to a different client. They are detached from the reality of themselves and just how wonderful and capable they are. Just as

I was. I needed that bucket of reality dumped on my head not just so I could see the survival adaptations that had made me sick. I needed to wake up so I could see myself as I really was, including all the good things.

This contradiction, then, seems obvious when you look in from the outside, but it is not clear to those with childhood trauma. Before we do this work, my clients, like many people with this kind of trauma, believe they are far from wonderful or capable. They do not register their successes as successes. They feel like they're failing. They believe they've got it all wrong. They feel shame instead of self-esteem. It is heart-breaking, perplexing and unfair.

The contradiction stems from their wounding and the survival adaptations they've developed to try and cope with it. Their unresolved trauma has left them carrying deeply untrue beliefs about themselves. Part of them believes they are not enough, that they are not doing enough, that they are broken, that they are failing, that they are damaged. Along with these beliefs, they will also feel intensely ashamed, afraid, terrified, sad, alone or angry. But in response to this pain they move further into their survival adaptations to try and cope.

Awareness of the contradiction is often people's wake-up call. As one client said to me:

How can I have so much in my life and still feel like a piece of shit? I give up, I really give up. I kept on going thinking one day I'd feel proud of myself, but it just gets worse and worse. I feel like I'm going mad because I look normal and have to pretend to be normal, but inside I'm a mess.

Unresolved trauma creates an internal experience of contradiction and conflict. When we're triggered, our wounding
makes us feel like *a piece of shit* and our survival adaptations
subconsciously move us into avoidance by pushing us to do
more, work harder, be better, figure it out. In response to the
sense of failure, worthlessness or low self-esteem, we subconsciously (and often obsessively and with a complete fixation)
focus on a specific solution that is not actually a solution at all.
This internal contradiction and conflict is the trauma.

Over time, this contradiction pushes us to extremes as we
either respond *from* our wounding, making life choices from
the baseline of 'I'm a piece of shit', or react *to* our wounding,
trying to prove it wrong. Either way, the inner conflict subconsciously controls our lives and decisions.

I often say to clients, and remind myself daily, that trauma
leaves us oscillating wildly between living in the fast lane of
the motorway (pushing, doing, proving, running at 100 miles
an hour) to crashing into the hard shoulder (strung out,
burned out, ashamed, in collapse). Trauma healing, then,
is about learning to live life in the middle lane – moderate,
manageable, realistic.

The first time I heard the analogy about the motorway
I found it confusing and depressing. I wanted to run in the fast
lane. I thought this was where successful people spent their
time. Challenging this perception, and learning that success
is not contingent on me pushing myself to death (and then
crashing), has been a huge shift. It wasn't something I could
really understand, or get behind, until I started to experience
how much better life was when I moved out of extremes and
into balance.

Know it all

As well as being phenomenally excellent humans, many of my clients also know a great deal about self-help and wellness. They know a lot of tools, they're well versed on the benefits of cold-water plunges. They can explain narcissism better than many psychologists I know. In short, my clients have achieved a lot *and* they know a lot.

This isn't a coincidence. *Figuring it all out* is an adaptation driven by their wounding. As our wounding shouts, 'You're failing, you're getting it wrong, you're worthless,' our survival adaptations activate to respond to the threat posed by not knowing or making a mistake.

We learn *all the things* because not knowing all the things feels deeply threatening. If we don't know, we move back into our wounding and feel as if we're failing. So we keep intellectualising and trying to figure it all out, running from the sense of failure or not-enoughness. We collect self-help books and tools and techniques. Our mind gets fuller and fuller. At times, knowing brings relief – we feel in control. But it can also bring a sense of confusion, overwhelm, shame or despair because we 'know everything' but are still in pain and struggling.

Working with my clients, who know so much but are still profoundly stuck, has helped me truly understand unconscious autopilot. My clients (and me BD) are stuck in their minds and literally unable to act. They want to heal but they cannot take action because taking action requires them to a) deviate from their neural survival map and do things differently and b) be in their bodies and connect to things they've been avoiding. And, without realising it, these are two things they've been running from.

We know we must heal, but we're subconsciously trying to do so in a way that avoids deviating from what is familiar and comfortable (overthinking) and moving towards the unfamiliar and dangerous (feeling). We want to keep learning and keep talking. We want to do anything and everything except feel or truly change. We desperately, urgently want to be well, but are unable to take meaningful action.

If this sounds a lot like the freeze response, that's because it is. So many of my clients are stuck in freeze with very little awareness that they're frozen – one foot on the accelerator and one on the brake. It's a very difficult, fairly abstract thing to get our heads around. Often we only see and feel just how frozen we have been as we begin to experience life in flow. The contrast teaches us where we need to head. Just as we have to experience The Solution before we really get it, our understanding of The Problem is also experiential. Reading about freeze is interesting, but truly understanding your own freeze state requires a level of conscious awareness and connection to your body that you may not yet have.

Trauma healing requires us to learn through experience. Reading this book will give you knowledge about both the problem you face and the solution, but healing requires moving slowly into awareness and action. This book is a call to action, but it's a message I make tentatively and respectfully. You must act, but it must also feel gentle. Too much change, too much feeling, too much of anything is still too much.

Inconsistency: A note on freedom

Pretty much every week for the past two years I've written an email newsletter called Notes on Freedom. It's a weekly email series containing 'easily digestible morsels of info on relational trauma and how to find freedom from it'. Literally, this is the tagline.

Admittedly, writing this very book has meant I've had to pause these emails to ensure my head doesn't explode, but nonetheless there has been a very satisfying consistency to the Notes. This consistency has been hard-won – it's something I've had to learn and practise over the years.

The Note I wrote on inconsistency is one of the highest viewed pages on my website. It's interesting, I think, that this *easily digestible morsel* has caught people's attention. It highlights that inconsistency, as a consequence of childhood trauma, is something we need to look at more closely. Rather than re-word something that's clearly resonating with thousands of people, I thought I'd just include it here for you:

Relational trauma and nervous system dysregulation go hand in hand. Dysregulation comes in many forms, but it always involves an overactive fight-flight-freeze response.

Often we operate within high arousal (anxiety, adrenaline, stress, reactivity, impulsivity, overexcitement). 'Switching off' is hard, particularly because we have a subconscious biological and psychological desire to maintain the go-go-go energy. So when we do 'stop', we're actually still going (scrolling on our phones, compulsively eating, picking our nails, tapping our feet). Until, eventually, we can't keep going any longer and we move into collapse and burnout.

Have you ever given much thought to what consistency actually is? Consistency is all about balance and rhythm. It's about regularity and flow – reliable, predictable.

Because the nervous system is the foundation of our entire being, when it is out of sync everything feels out of sync. When it is unbalanced, we are unbalanced. When it is inconsistent, we are inconsistent.

When our nervous system only operates at full throttle or in collapse, we too are yanked between these extremes. Finding long-term balance and consistency in our daily routine, exercise, food, relationships, health or work feels painfully hard to achieve.

At times in my life I have felt deep shame about my inability to be consistent. I've heard many others around me voice this shame too. But, and I say this with complete conviction: we have nothing to be ashamed of.

It is not lack of willpower, lack of ambition or lack of discipline that leads to inconsistency. Our bodies and minds are overwhelmed and out of balance. Not because of anything we did (or didn't) do, but because of what those around us did (or did not) do many years ago.

For you and me, freedom from inconsistency comes as we refocus on our trauma healing, for this is where the real magic happens. Freedom and consistency come as we learn to self-regulate.

Inconsistency is debilitating and shaming. We feel *less than* because we struggle to do the thing we want to do when we said we'd do it. There's so much judgement, so much 'come on, pull your socks up' directed at those who struggle to move into consistency and regularity.

Although I can't stop your grandfather/mother/partner raising an eyebrow when you don't meet their expectations, I hope that this explanation will ignite just a little more of your own self-compassion around this. Inconsistency and extremes are hardwired into your nervous system, but this book will teach you how to begin to re-wire so you can move into the consistency and rhythm you crave and need.

Deprivation

'The muffin' is still my favourite example of how bizarre, remarkable and painfully efficient trauma responses are.

Just after the release of my first book I was on a podcast, and the host told me that for years he couldn't go into certain coffee shops. He'd walk up to the counter and instantly feel uncomfortable, stressed and dissociated. Over time, once he'd started on his own journey of trauma healing, he realised that the muffins on the coffee shop counter had been triggering a trauma response. This poor guy, who just wanted a morning coffee, was flooded by shame and fear at the mere sight and smell of a muffin.

Once you hear his story it makes sense. His mother, who was emotionally abusive, used to serve muffins every Saturday morning. Along with the muffin came shaming, criticism and cruelty. His nervous system was picking up on the imprint of this trauma (the smell and sight of the muffin) and triggered his old traumatic reaction (freeze) and survival adaptation (avoidance – leave, now). It did this to keep him safe, but safe in this instance meant 'away from the muffin'.

This example is fantastic, I think. It helps us all see that although our nervous system aims to keep us safe, it creates unnerving experiences that don't make logical sense in adult life. It can also keep us away from things in life that not only pose no threat, but that are also really rather lovely (like a muffin).

Trauma can lead us away from so much that could feel good and bring joy into our lives. It can keep us away from new experiences, holidays, socialising, relationships, new opportunities, touch and love. It's not just about missing out on muffins; it's about unknowingly and unconsciously moving away from the things we need and deserve.

My clients are all in various states of deprivation caused by their triggered reactions. They want connection and friendship. They want to travel. They want a new career. They want a new type of relationship. They want to start a new hobby. They want something *different* for themselves, something better. But as they move towards these things (whether it's a muffin, celebrating their birthday, a third date or coffee with a new friend) they're triggered and pulled back into an old reaction. Their neural map wants to keep them away from these things to keep them safe, because in childhood they were somehow connected to threat, overwhelm and emotional pain.

This is one of the most unfair consequences of childhood trauma, because so much of what we avoid are the things we need to heal us. Moving towards healthy things that we want and need is part of recovery – part of this new, different life we build as we heal our trauma. But we do this oh so slowly. Gradually, with the speed of a sloth and in a wholly new way, we move towards them. Slow and steady, aware and connected to our body and our feelings, is how we widen our window of tolerance and over time, become able to eat the muffin. To learn more about the window of tolerance, see page 142.

Relationship pain

The disconnection we can experience in relationships is one of the most painful outcomes of trauma. The muffin story shows that triggers (things connected to the imprint) really can be anything, but because childhood trauma is primarily caused by traumatic experiences within relationships, the trigger is often *relational*. Our triggers are often to do with other people and our sense of security in relation to them.

Some common triggers that can activate our wounding are:

- Making a mistake or thinking we have made a mistake within the relationship/social group
- Conflict
- Feeling disliked/hated
- Being excluded or feeling excluded
- Feeling rejected
- Feeling abandoned
- Being criticised or feeling criticised
- Feeling like we've let someone down or upset them
- Someone ignoring our boundary
- Someone setting a healthy boundary
- Appropriate vulnerability, dependence and neediness
- Appropriate emotional connection
- Socialising/groups
- Compliments and/or a sense of other people's expectations
- Sex, touch and cuddling.

The experiences I've listed are common to all relationships. There's nothing objectively unusual about the situations, emotions and dynamics I've described. In small doses, they're all facets of *normal* relationships. All relationships involve people making mistakes; all relationships involve conflict. Even being disliked, not invited or criticised are normal (albeit unpleasant) parts of human relationships and social groups.

Although those of us with childhood trauma might read this list and baulk, those without childhood trauma can read this list and think, 'what's the big deal?' They can respond with neutrality because, although they've most likely experienced everything on this list at one time or another, similar experiences in childhood were not traumatic for them. They did not find these childhood experiences overwhelmingly threatening, most likely because they subconsciously knew they had the internal (e.g. self-belief) and external (e.g. support) resources they needed to cope with these experiences.

Those who grew up securely attached, regulated, connected and feeling safe can experience rejection, say, and navigate the painful experience without moving into an old survival response because they have no wounding caused by rejection. For those with childhood trauma, the normal 'downs' of relationships feel deeply threatening because in childhood we experienced these things in a way that felt unsafe and too much for us. Rejection, criticism, conflict, boundary violations and so on were traumatic experiences, so as adults today, even healthy relationships can feel profoundly painful and confusing because they are god-awful reminders of past threats that trigger the old reaction.

My clients have all experienced intense, painful triggered reactions within relationships, as have I. Often these happen within close relationships, but any and all interactions with other humans can contain reminders of our wounding and trigger a strong survival response. Think of Sophia, who I spoke of in the last chapter. She was strongly and intensely triggered by Nick's dismissive tone of voice. This wasn't a close relationship, nor was it one Sophia was invested in or particularly cared about. Nonetheless, it activated her childhood wounding and prevented her from showing up as her grounded, regulated, adult self.

The common relational triggers I've listed above look obvious when they're written down, but in real life they're extremely hard to see and separate from. In real life, recognising your relational triggers is not a clear-cut, obvious process. It takes time to see and feel our activation because in real time our reactions feel appropriate and warranted. Standing back and seeing that our wounding and survival response has been activated is extremely hard, so when we do get the fleeting sense that the reaction is *old* it's a big win.

Recently, a wonderful client of mine, Steph, came to a session distressed and frustrated because she'd spent two days flooded by an old trauma response. Steph had been in a state of chronic anxiety and stress, shame, panic, rumination (uncontrollable overthinking) and compulsive eating. She'd been triggered by an acquaintance turning away from her as she tried to say hi. Initially she was embarrassed and flustered, but soon she spiralled into an intense old reaction. She felt overwhelmingly conflicted and torn. Even though her rational, adult self was saying, 'You've done nothing wrong, let it go, she was probably just in a bad mood,' her wounding flooded her with shame and despair, and the belief that she was bad and worthless. Her survival adaptations also kicked in. She was dissociated and thinking obsessively about how she could fix the situation. She composed and deleted multiple messages to the acquaintance. Eventually she sent a message unconsciously designed to flatter the person and repair a mistake she was certain she must have made – a fawn response. Her despair became overwhelming when they didn't reply to her message.

This experience was incredibly painful for Steph, but the pain wasn't *about* the adult relationship. Her adult self knew that the acquaintance's feelings towards her would have little bearing on her life; she knew she had done nothing wrong and she knew that the acquaintance was prone to being offish and grumpy. The pain was old and deep, belonging to a young part of herself that grew up with a mother who often became passive aggressive and gave Steph the silent treatment. The acquaintance's behaviour subsciously reminded Steph of her mother and how unsafe she felt in this formative relationship.

Trauma work, particularly at the start, is about untangling the spaghetti. We slow things down and pull the strands of the old trauma and the present situation apart. Childhood trauma leaves us unable to see the wood for the trees in relationships, so we act from our wounding and our survival adaptations and in doing so perpetuate the disconnection and pain. Instead of moving towards our pain and tending to it, we unknowingly operate from it. We scream at our partners, shame our children, anxiously pace, worry, pander to our friends, cancel plans, and blame and hate ourselves. On some level we know we're doing these things, but we're also on autopilot. We're frozen and stuck, feeling compelled to react the only way we know how.

Trauma healing is about slowing down so we can separate and see the truth of what's going on – so we can pull apart our old trauma from our adult relationships. As we do this, we connect to our agency, and become able to make a different choice and take a different action.

Emotional flashbacks

Survival adaptations often *feel* different from the way our wounding feels. At times, our adaptations can even feel good and powerful, but our wounding is vulnerable, in need and in pain. Most often when we're triggered in adult life, we move so quickly into the adaptation that we completely avoid the pain of our wounding. Sometimes, though, our wounding floods our system and we're thrown right back into all the old pain.

Because of this, I want to introduce you to the term *emotional flashback*. It's a term used by Pete Walker in his seminal book *Complex PTSD: From Surviving to Thriving*, and one that has been profoundly helpful for many of my clients. Pete Walker writes:

> Emotional flashbacks are sudden and often prolonged regressions to the overwhelming feeling-states of being abused/abandoned as a child. These feeling states can include overwhelming fear, shame, alienation, rage, grief and depression . . . Flashbacks can range in intensity from subtle to horrific. They can also vary in duration, ranging from moments to weeks.[1]

Unlike the flashbacks that accompany PTSD, complex trauma flashbacks do not have a visual or auditory component. Instead of images of the traumatic experience, our mind and body are flooded by the old emotions, sensations, thoughts and beliefs that we experienced at the time of the initial trauma.

Many find the term *emotional flashback* extremely helpful to describe the moments they're flooded by their wounding. A client of mine, Izzy, found the term helpful and descriptive following a triggered reaction she experienced early on in her healing journey. Izzy lived outside London but had caught the train into Kings Cross so she could attend a job interview. Like many with complex relational trauma, Izzy found travelling extremely stressful. As she sat on the train she felt highly anxious, unsafe and jittery. At times she couldn't catch her breath. This was made worse because she had a loop of 'You're a failure, you'll never get this job' playing in her mind.

Izzy cannot remember how the interview went, as she was dissociated and panicked. As she started her journey home she felt completely defeated. She was flooded by an intense sense of failure, by feelings of shame and an urge to disappear. She strongly felt that everyone in her life would be better off without her. She remembers putting her hands on her temples to try and switch off the incessant barrage of self-hate and shame her mind was spouting at her.

I spoke to Izzy the following day. When I used the term *emotional flashback* to describe what Izzy experienced following the interview she burst out crying.

Yes, that's what it was. I couldn't escape the feelings. I felt like I was drowning. This is how I felt all the time as a kid – like a failure, like I'd let everyone down. I just wanted out of everything – of my family and my body and life. I felt so scared yesterday because I haven't felt that way for so long.

The intensity of Izzy's emotional flashback was in part because of the stress she felt on the way to the interview. She was stressed, strung out and on edge before she even got there. She was already triggered, so the sense of failure she felt during the interview tipped her into intense despair and collapse. Simply hearing her experience named was extremely helpful for her, as it helped normalise and make sense of it.

If you cast your mind back over the past few months, can you recall a time when you were flooded in this way? When you were overrun by old beliefs and old emotions? Perhaps you too, like Izzy, will find comfort and resonance in the term *emotional flashback*. It comes to life as we start to use it, I think because it so perfectly describes the experiences of being flooded by our childhood wounding.

Disconnection from self

Childhood relational trauma damages our understanding of who we are. Our experiences leave us with painful, damaging beliefs that we are worthless, bad, invisible, too much, damaged, broken, disgusting or a failure. These beliefs are often buried, but subconsciously direct our thinking, behaviour and choices.

The beliefs and the shame, fear and anger are part of the traumatic reaction, but of course children don't know this. I mean, of course they don't – most adults don't know this. As children we cannot gain perspective and say to ourselves, 'Dad's triggered so he's being aggressive and controlling – it has nothing to do with me.' Instead we might self-blame, panic, act out, feel ashamed, reach for comfort food, feel confused, try to appease, try to be 'good' or simply shut down and hide. As we move into these nervous system-led ways of being, relating and coping, we disconnect from our true feelings and the present moment. We are no longer anchored into our body and our sense of self – regulated, open, connected and spontaneous. Instead we're in survival and doing what we *should do* or *have to do* to minimise, avoid or appease the threat, rather than being *ourselves*.

The process of growing up and becoming a human adult is all about adapting. We want children to understand that they don't, for example, swear at the headmaster or strip off in the supermarket. We teach, model and discipline, and they *adapt*. Adaptation is a normal part of becoming a well-functioning adult. But the adaptations we experience as part of a traumatic reaction are not like the normal adaptive process of growing up. Those we develop in response to chronic overwhelm, fear and shame do not lead to growth and flourishing. They are fear-led adaptations designed to avoid, protect and disconnect. They take us away from authenticity and into autopilot, away from presence and into performance. Because of the disconnection, we don't learn what we truly like or dislike. We don't learn what we truly value or want from life. We don't learn to operate from instinct (which requires us to feel our 'yes' and 'no' in our body). Likewise, as we disconnect from our body and true self, we disconnect from our passion and our purpose. Instead of present, open, connected, authentic, we operate from a neural survival map. We are trauma-led instead of self-led.

Disconnection from self also causes boundary issues. Boundaries are our limits – they're what we will and will not tolerate and accept. They create our comfort zone – a sacred container that enables us to feel safe and comfortable, and have self-respect and self-esteem.[2] They're highly personal, and link to and define our values and identity. Knowing our limits requires us to know ourselves. Given that trauma disconnects us from our self, it is inevitable that those with childhood trauma struggle with boundaries (self-led limits).

Boundaries are a weird concept. Those with boundaries don't really understand why those of us who struggle with boundaries go on about them. To them, those invisible limits that link to their sturdy sense of self are as natural as breathing. To us, these invisible limits are fascinating and intimidating because we're aware we somehow have an issue with them. It can be hard to imagine how we might use them. Getting our head around boundaries takes time. As we connect back to our self, we become consciously aware of our own limits, just as we become aware of our preferences. We also become consciously aware of other people's boundaries. We learn to see and feel when we are overstepping someone else's limits. Over time, we re-establish respect for ourselves and others.

Trauma healing is about learning *how* to re-anchor back into self. As we interrupt our trauma-led patterns and build capacity, we reconnect to our true self. As we do, we come to know our preferences *and* our limits – we get clear on who we are. Authenticity replaces autopilot.

Familiar is comfortable

Trauma has us repeating and repeating old protective reactions, and as we do, the neural pathways supporting the protective reactions embed more and more. One explanation for this is that humans are hardwired to become hardwired, so it's very easy to wind up repeating maladaptive patterns; there are also other reasons we repeat and repeat. To illustrate these other reasons, I'm going to tell you about one of my first clients, Annie.

Annie grew up with an alcoholic father. He was emotionally volatile and often verbally abusive to Annie and her mother. Annie's mother was highly anxious, and to cope, she kept compulsively busy.

To escape her childhood home, Annie married John when she was 22. John drank a lot, and was unpredictable and often verbally abusive. Despite this, Annie had two children with him. John and Annie divorced when Annie was 28, and Annie went to live with her mother's sister, who she'd always had a good relationship with. Her aunt helped Annie with the children, and supported her in returning to work. After about 18 months, Annie and her children moved into a nice apartment. Things felt good and solid for the first time in long time. Annie met Martin about nine months later. They took the relationship slowly, and things appeared to be going well. There were some red flags, though – he drank heavily at the weekends and as a result often became angry and depressed.

Despite the red flags – or in fact, *because* of the red flags that subconsciously drew Annie to Martin – they moved in together. This four-year relationship was abusive and traumatic. Once the relationship ended and Annie was trying to rebuild her life, she truly understood, for the first time, that her traumatic childhood was repeating and repeating. She was seeking out the familiar, even though it was destructive and damaging. Even though living with John and then Martin had been painful, to Annie it was familiar. She had instigated beautiful change in her life, then undermined her success by seeking out old, familiar situations and relationships.

Eighty per cent of my clients work in dysfunctional, toxic, stressful work environments. This 80 per cent also grew up in highly stressful homes. They've learned to function, even excel, in high-stress environments. They're used to working in the fast lane, and they associate success with pain and stress. To my clients (and to me before I was diagnosed), work and success are supposed to hurt. This is what their mind, body and soul know to be true based on their childhood experiences. They're hardwired to try harder because as children they didn't receive the implicit message, 'Stop now darling; that is enough, you've done well enough, *you* are enough.' Now that they are adults, their wounding tells them they're not enough, and they need to try harder, so they react to it and keep on pushing. And by *they*, obviously, I also mean me.

All humans are subconsciously attracted to people, situations and energy that feel familiar, as Annie was. This works very well for those who grew up in calm, secure homes, as they're likely to seek out something equally lovely. But for those with unresolved childhood trauma, it means we're frequently (and outside of conscious awareness) attracted to something with a sting in the tail. We move towards what we know: stress, chaos, dysfunction, emotional disconnection or worse. Not only do we move towards dysregulation, we unconsciously *create* it via our thinking, emotions, sensations and behaviours.

Our wounding and survival adaptations feel right and comfortable because they're all we know. This sense of comfort has a lot to do with things being predictable. Predictably painful, yes, but predictable none the less. So weirdly, we feel in control.

As well as the basic idea that we're attracted to what's familiar, many trauma practitioners believe we subconsciously *recreate* the same situation to give ourselves the opportunity to respond in the way we needed to and wanted to in childhood. This idea is based on the incomplete survival response that trauma creates.

Because during the initial experience our survival response is set off but not mobilised and resolved (so, we can't run or fight, for example), we move into a prolonged traumatic reaction. Healing, then, is about finding or creating *resolution*. And one way to do this is to repeat the original trauma, right? Annie repeated close relationships with male alcoholics. As dysfunctional and painful as this is, the third repetition pierced through Annie's conscious awareness. It woke her up and showed her that there was unresolved trauma that needed her attention. My clients repeatedly find themselves in highly stressful work environments, and again, as painful as this re-enactment process is, once we can see the repetition, we can do the work needed to create resolution, rather than continued repetition. Awareness of repetition is unpleasant, but it can also be the wake-up call we greatly need.

Neuroplasticity: The cons

The neural pathways that move you into survival at any sign of threat become stronger and more ingrained over time. These pathways are designed to protect us, but they lead to imbalance internally and in our life. All my clients tell me they feel simultaneously stuck and out of control. There's a contradiction here that only makes sense once you look through a trauma framework. They feel stuck because they're repeating old reactions (and are therefore experiencing the same outcomes). They feel out of control because neuroplasticity has ensured that their trauma response is automatic (and therefore happening largely outside of their conscious awareness).

Neuroplasticity refers to the lifelong capacity of the brain, and the entire nervous system, to rewire itself in response to experiences. 'Neuro' refers to neurons – the nerve cells that are the building blocks of the nervous system. Plasticity refers to the cells' malleability and ability to change. The nervous system has evolved to learn, remember and repeat.

Synapses are the microscopic gaps between neurons where messages are relayed. As we move through life and have different or repeated experiences, some connections are strengthened while others are weakened. This process is called synaptic pruning.

Neurons that are used frequently develop stronger synaptic connections and pathways. Neurons that are rarely or never used become weaker or are eliminated. The power of neuro-plasticity is how we become so profoundly, unconsciously stuck in our trauma responses over time. Don't panic, though, because neuroplasticity is also the power that will get you unstuck and move you into healing.

I recently started working with Dan, who is 33 years old and feels completely stuck, because he is. He feels out of control, because he is. Here is what he told me:

I feel like a failure because I don't do anything. I drop the kids off at school and then do nothing. Years are just passing by.

My anxiety no longer makes any sense at all. I'm just anxious all the time. Whether I'm trying to decide what to cook for dinner or just waking up in the morning . . . it's there. I can't stop it or make it ease up at all.

Although there's nothing objectively terrifying in Dan's life, he is terrified. This imprint of fear started when Dan was about five years old and his father left and never came back. The old fear pushes Dan into anxiety *and* avoidance, as he subconsciously avoids things that feel unsafe. This tendency to avoid as a way to try to manage the fear and anxiety compounded and became stronger and more intense until he dropped out of university at 19. Today, Dan cannot work and struggles to leave the house. Dan's life has become smaller and smaller as his nervous system has wired itself to focus on survival.

The point I'm trying to make here is that trauma responses become stronger and more automatic over time. It's almost as if our survival programming takes on a life of its own. Our nervous system, fuelled by the astonishing power of neuroplasticity, strengthens our neural survival map and weakens our neural safety map (the neural pathways that search for signs of safety, comfort and ease). What can feel like a choice in our 20s can feel disturbingly compulsive and automatic in our 40s.

Neuroplasticity is self-led. It belongs to you. It's a powerful force that exists within your body. Your nervous system didn't need a doctor or a specialist to teach it how to build its survival map, and your nervous system doesn't need a specialist to teach it to wire itself differently. Over time, as you practise a new way of being and relating, neuroplasticity will respond by creating a whole new map.

Addictive processes

My first book, *You're Not Broken*, talks extensively about why so many people with childhood trauma become locked into addictive processes as a way to mitigate, avoid and cope with their pain. So I'm not going to go into too much detail here. This isn't just because I don't want to repeat the same content. It's because I know you're already aware that many of us seamlessly move from trauma into addiction. As I describe in the previous chapter (see page 67), addictions are simply another type of survival adaption. They aren't pathological, they're protective.

Every client that walks through my door has become stuck in their survival adaptation – the adaptations have, in many ways, become an addictive process. I say 'every' because this isn't just about substance addiction. Nor is it just about those intense process addictions we all recognise as addictive and highly problematic such as bulimia or gambling. I do work with men and women who are stuck in these kinds of process addictions, or substance addictions to substances including cocaine, alcohol or prescription meds. But more often I work with those who are locked into much more subtle addictive processes. This subtlety, combined with how socially accept-able the addictive processes are, makes it very difficult for clients to acknowledge their stuckness.

Here I'm thinking about compulsive processes and behav-iours like overthinking, worry and rumination, creating/moving into chaos and intensity, work, phone use, busyness, planning, people-pleasing. These more subtle addictive processes are linked to different aspects of the survival response. Take over-thinking, worry and rumination, which are, of course, cognitive manifestations of anxious, adrenalised flight energy. Over time, thanks to neuroplasticity (see pages 93–5), these compulsive processes become habitual and hardwired.

Sure, we don't get hooked into these ways of being in quite the same way as we might to cocaine, say. But we do become subconsciously reliant on the process to help us navigate and survive our inner wounding and outer world. In reality, any survival adaptation can become part of an addictive process.

As is the case with any aspect of our trauma patterning, seeing and acknowledging the lack of control and choice we now have around these kinds of behaviours and processes is an essential first step to breaking the habit.

Toxic stress and the body

I've already mentioned the ground-breaking research on the impact of Adverse Childhood Experiences (ACEs) on long-term health. This research demonstrates that experiences like neglect, abuse and household dysfunction contribute to long-term health issues like cardiovascular disease, cancer and autoimmune issues. Here, I'm going to give you a little more detail about what these studies have uncovered. I'm also going to explain the follow-up research into precisely *how* childhood trauma affects our physical health. Because understanding the physiological mechanisms that lead from traumatic childhood experience to long-term health issues is essential if we want to know how to heal.

The first major ACE study looked at the relationship between the number of ACEs reported by more than 17,000 individuals in the USA and their long-term health. It found that the more ACEs individuals reported, the greater their risks of health-harming behaviours, such as heavy drinking, smoking or sexual risk-taking, and both infectious and chronic diseases.[3] As the world has woken up to the importance of these findings, and the measurement of ACEs has been standardised, these findings have been replicated worldwide across many different countries and groups of people. For a list of ACEs see Appendix A.

In 2017, Professor Karen Hughes and her colleagues published a systematic review and meta-analysis of all the ACE research to date. They examined 37 studies with a total of 253,719 participants and found that individuals who had experienced four or more ACEs were at an increased risk of all 23 poor health outcomes.[4] These include:

- Obesity
- Diabetes
- Cardiovascular disease
- Cancer
- Liver or digestive disease
- Respiratory disease
- Anxiety
- Suicide attempt
- Mental ill health
- Drug or alcohol misuse
- Self-harm.

Meta-analyses are very robust. They're the research equivalent of a mic-drop. They play a pivotal role in moving something from theory to fact. It is now wholly true to say that experiencing multiple ACEs in childhood is a major risk factor for many health conditions. There's no wriggle room here. It just is what it is.

As robust as this research is, Hughes and her colleagues only focused on the 23 most common specific health outcomes. This means that many poor health outcomes are not included. Other research demonstrates the link between ACEs and auto-immune issues, chronic fatigue, multiple sclerosis, psoriasis, chronic obstructive pulmonary disease (COPD), migraines and inflammatory bowel disease (IBS).[5]

The mounting evidence of the relationship between ACEs and ill health leads the worldwide research community to the much harder task of trying to explain what's actually going on. Why does childhood stress and trauma put us at major risk of long-term health issues? What's actually happening in the body to move us from trauma to ill health?

Stress is the simple answer. But in the early 2000s, Harvard's Center on the Developing Child coined the term *toxic stress* to describe the excessive stress response associated with trauma and early-life stress.[6] The type of stress associated with childhood trauma is not the same as the normal, adaptive stress that we may think of when we hear the word 'stress'. This isn't 'Oh how irritating, I just missed the bus.' This is something chemically very different. It's toxic, literally. Harvard's Center on the Developing Child writes:

The introduction of the term *toxic stress* reflects extensive scientific knowledge about the effects of excessive activation of stress response systems on a child's developing brain, as well as the immune system, metabolic regulatory systems, and cardiovascular system. Experiencing ACEs triggers all of these interacting stress response systems. When a child experiences multiple ACEs over time – especially without supportive relationships with adults to provide buffering protection – the experiences will trigger an excessive and long-lasting stress response, which can have a wear-and-tear effect on the body, like revving a car engine for days or weeks at a time.

We're also beginning to be able to explain what toxic stress is physiologically. Biological indicators of toxic stress are inflammation, shortened telomeres (these are 'caps' on the ends of your chromosomes, which carry genetic information in your cells, and are notably shorter in those with high ACE scores) and an accumulation of stress hormones. It's not ordinary stress, which can be healthy when appropriate. It's chronic, excessive activation and dysregulation of multiple, interwoven stress response systems that lead to biological changes and, over time, disease.[7]

As *ugh* as all this might sound, this information can be used to empower – it can, if we allow it, lead us into agency and action. Now we know toxic stress is *the problem*, we can learn how to reduce and reverse it. This is precisely what the tools in this book are designed to help you do. As you move into self-led action and integrate the four core capacities, you can slowly de-activate your stress response systems, re-regulate your nervous system and move into healing and health.

Self-reliance

Before we move on, I need to highlight that a common consequence of childhood trauma is extreme self-reliance. Admittedly, trauma can also predispose us to extreme neediness and over-reliance on other people too, but here I want to focus on the common trauma-led need to figure out everything *alone*. We do not ask for help. We do not share our needs or pain. Or rather, we *cannot* ask for help and we *cannot* share our needs or pain. We cannot do these things because we have little experience of other people as a source of healthy support. Our role models in childhood may have been intensely self-reliant and/or emotionally unavailable. Or, worse, the adults in our lives may have been abusive or neglectful, which taught us that not only are other people unable to support us, but also that they are not safe. To cope, we adapt – we learn to zip up our needs and pain and rely only on ourselves.

But we're social animals. Optimal human functioning happens when we're part of a healthy tribe – when we can connect, share, support and, yes, rely on others. Connection is the key concept here. Relational trauma moves us into patterns of disconnection in relationships. Trauma healing is about reconnecting in a healthy, new way to others. We connect to others not *because* we're unwell, but because we're human. It took me a long time to understand that asking for support and sharing my fears wasn't something I had to do because I was broken and unwell, but because I was human. Allowing ourselves to share our emotional pain and receive support is the top of the mountain we're trying to reach. Healthy, functional adults can ask for support, reassurance and validation from other healthy, functional adults when they're in need. This is not a sign of radical dysfunction and trauma, it's a sign of wellness. Asking for help, sharing our deepest fears or simply allowing another to help us are not just signs of trauma healing, they're signs we're moving into thriving.

I hope you can begin to move towards the truth. Sharing our feelings and asking for support feels intensely risky because in the past this healthy, beautiful move towards connection was rejected. It was not an emotionally safe thing to do. Because of this, it's feasible you've built friendships and connections that cannot facilitate vulnerability and support. Over time, this will change and soften. It won't feel comfortable, but slowly, and in your own time, you'll move towards authentic connection and support. This could be a triggering thought, but I'm saying this because for a long time I thought trauma healing meant that one day I would no longer need to share my fears and pain with others – that one day I'd be completely self-reliant. Now I know that healthy, functional and healed involves more vulnerability and support, not less.

The concept of self-led healing may have felt appealing to the parts of you that carry those old beliefs – the belief you must do this alone, that others can't be trusted, that vulnerability is dangerous or that asking for support is weak. If the appeal of self-reliance got you here, great. Just know that although self-led trauma healing builds healthy resilience and self-connection, over time it also builds healthy interdependence and other-connection. If the image of healthy interdependence with others feels too much right now, let it float away from your awareness. You don't have to think about or action this right now.

For now, just begin to get curious about the fact that the urgent pull you may have to figure all this out alone, the mistrust you may feel towards others, and the deep discomfort you may feel towards healthy interdependence, may not be an adult choice. It's more likely that these things are a consequence of childhood trauma, and therefore part of the autopilot and adaptations you'll slowly move out of.

A pause

To be honest, writing the past few chapters felt unexpectedly hard. As I wrote my first book I revelled in the intellectual explanations of trauma – I loved looking at it, turning it upside down and figuring it out (sigh). But this time I've been aware of my own resistance to being in *the problem* – a kind of energetic pull towards something lighter and brighter. I can feel my body relax and my energy flow as I move into the next part of the book. What a joy and a privilege it is to now share with you *the solution*.

Part 2

The solution

Chapter Four

How to heal your trauma

This chapter is all about how to heal your trauma. Here, I explain what you're aiming for and how to get there (although admittedly this 'how to' piece won't be complete until you've read the whole book).

As you know by now, I have come to believe that trauma healing happens as we learn to safely, gently and courageously take action. I believe that therapy alone cannot heal childhood trauma, but that therapy coupled with self-led action will create profound, deep healing. This chapter is where I begin to turn this statement into a program of healing, as I explain the four capacities of trauma healing: signalling safety, awareness, connection to our adult self and self-led action.

This chapter may not always feel comfortable, but the truths it contains will help you heal your trauma by reclaiming your agency and taking action, one day at a time.

The mountain top

Before I start, I want to highlight a challenge we all face. Because not only are those with childhood trauma frequently triggered and pulled into an old survival adaptation, but unlike those who do *not* have this kind trauma, we have little experience of a regulated equilibrium to return to. We react strongly to something that happens in our lives but we have no awareness of our body's regulated state, so we don't know where we need to return to afterwards.

A good analogy is expecting someone lost in a dense forest at the bottom of a deep mountain valley, who has no map or compass and has never seen or heard of the sacred place at the top of the mountain, to find their way there.

This describes all my clients when they first start working with me – trying to find their way out of a forest to a sacred mountain top that they've never previously seen or heard of. They have no *embodied understanding* of what they're seeking and no sense of how to find their way there. So much of my work is about teaching people how to find their way to the mountain top and how to recognise this sacred place when they arrive.

The emergence of self

Diagram 2 *is* the mountain top. It's the sacred place that you can, and will, reach as you begin to reclaim your agency and take self-led action. I hope that although this diagram is new, it also feels *right*. It shows you where you're heading – this is healing. Or, perhaps, this is *healed*.

As we move out of physiological survival and into safety – a sense of openness, ease, comfort, balance, release, connection,

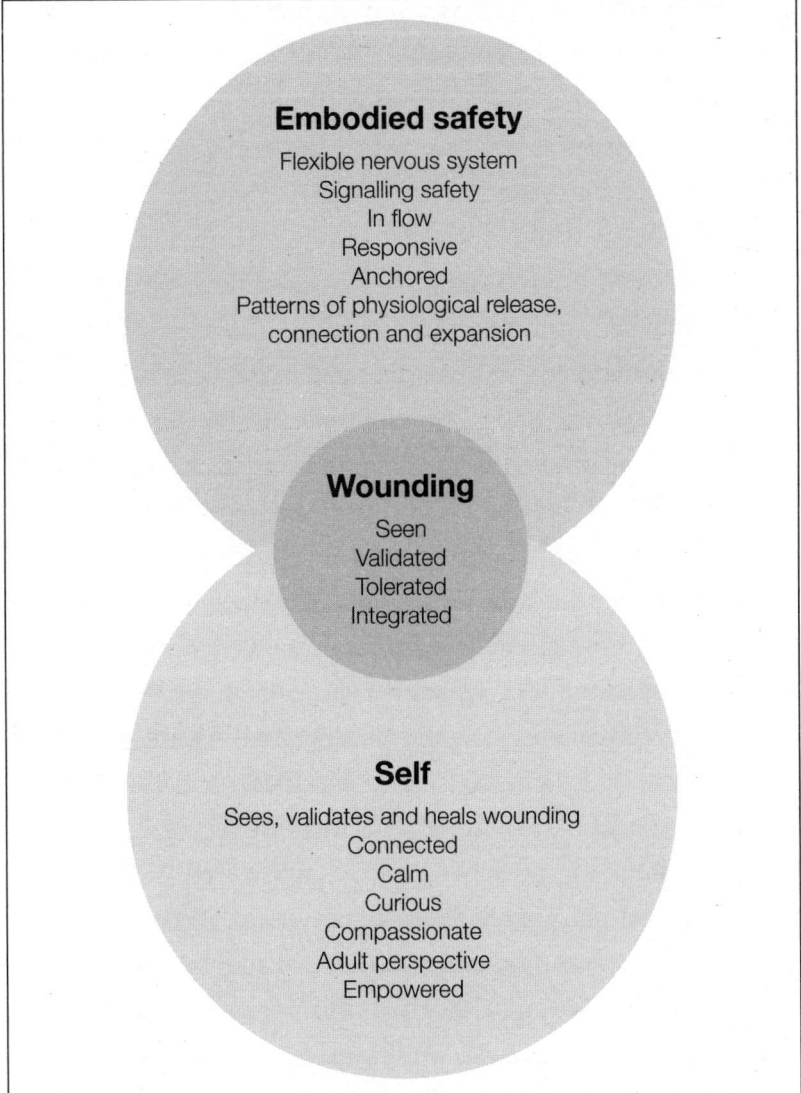

Embodied safety
Flexible nervous system
Signalling safety
In flow
Responsive
Anchored
Patterns of physiological release,
connection and expansion

Wounding
Seen
Validated
Tolerated
Integrated

Self
Sees, validates and heals wounding
Connected
Calm
Curious
Compassionate
Adult perspective
Empowered

Diagram 2: Childhood trauma healing: The sacred mountain top

As we increasingly take action to signal safety to our nervous system and move into regulation, our sense of self emerges – consciously aware, present, curious, compassionate, empowered and with an adult perspective. When this happens, we can separate from, see and validate our wounding, which helps us heal and move into connection with our sense of agency and choice.

expansion, regulation, flow and movement in our bodies, emotions and minds, something quite magical happens. We discover self. For many of those with childhood trauma who feel wildly disconnected from who they *really* are, this reconnection is life changing.

This process is also unnervingly simple. As we reconnect to self, we realise we've spent our lives unnecessarily chasing a false ideal. We don't need to search for an identity that has been lost or damaged. We simply need to pause and step back, out of the trauma and dysregulation. As we reconnect, we realise self was always there. To read more about the connection between self-regulation and self, see page 184.

Self emerges as we pause and reconnect to the present moment and our body. It is our regulated state, which we move towards as we signal safety to our nervous system. It is our seat of conscious awareness, which we discover as we separate and observe ourselves. It is our wise, compassionate adult self, which can respond with perspective and kindness. It is our sense of empowered agency, which we reclaim as we reconnect.

Our regulated, present, adult, empowered self has the power to heal us. There's no real mystery to it. Self heals our trauma – our wounding and our survival adaptations – simply by being *self*. As we signal safety to our nervous system, release and regulate, we heal. As we're able to feel and release our trauma in a safe, contained way, we heal. As we are curious about, and present with, our trauma, we heal. As we separate from and see our trauma with an adult perspective, we heal. As we respond to our trauma with compassion, we heal. And as we act from self, not from trauma and autopilot, we heal.

The way I teach self-led trauma healing is structured and clear. I break things down so that you can easily move into action. But despite all you're about to read about daily action, capacities, tools and principles, I don't want you to lose sight of the magic, the soul and the importance of what you're doing. Because what you're doing is reconnecting to, and reclaiming, your self. What you're doing, as you reclaim your agency and unlock your power to self-heal, is nothing short of miraculous.

Symbiosis

The concepts and theories I include in this chapter do not belong to me. Arguably, they don't *belong* to anyone, but I want to explain the lineage of what I'm presenting, because currently, leading therapeutic approaches are all urging us in the same direction.

Polyvagal Theory, described by Dr Stephen Porges, and Somatic Experiencing (SE), a trauma treatment created by Dr Peter Levine that focuses on releasing trauma energy from the body, have illustrated that trauma healing goes hand in hand with regulating, and signalling safety to, the nervous system. From these somatic (body-based) approaches we've gained clarity about the pivotal role of the ventral vagal nerve in nervous system regulation. We've also come to understand that presence, curiosity and compassion are more available to us when this nerve is activated.

The somatic approaches, then, are urging us to regulate our nervous systems so we can become present and connect to our curiosity and compassion. Internal Family Systems (IFS), a leading therapeutic model for working with childhood trauma, urges us to understand this presence, curiosity and compassion as Self. Frank Anderson, a leading IFS practitioner and educator, writes:

The Self is the core of psychic balance, the seat of consciousness and inner source of love. Everyone has Self. Just as light can be both particle and wave, the Self can show up in the energy of certain feeling states (curiosity, calm, courage, compassion, love) or with the sense of an individual being present.[1]

Stephen Porges' Polyvagal Theory, Peter Levine's Somatic Experiencing and Richard Schwartz's Internal Family Systems all fit together and work in harmony with each other. Gabor Maté's Compassionate Inquiry and Bessel Van Der Kolk's well known therapeutic approach also support the same thesis.

This symbiosis is helping these modalities gain traction and moving the whole field forward. Although some people are irritated by the current inescapable dominance of 'the trauma kings',[2] their theories have also created a powerful shift in how we approach mental health. Many of the concepts, terms and principles I'm presenting here stem from these approaches. As I do in my practice, I'm weaving the polyvagal approach and the IFS approach together to create an accessible, self-led way-in to trauma healing. Just as 'the kings of trauma' have built their approaches on the phenomenal practitioners that went before them (such as Moshé Feldenkrais, Pia Mellody, Francine Shapiro, Stanley Rosenberg, Janina Fisher and Babette Rothschild), so am I.

Capacity building

Trauma healing is an active process. It has to be, because inaction (freeze, stuckness, repetition, patterning, autopilot) *is* the problem. As I've said (and am probably going to say approximately another 400 times before we're done): to heal we have to slowly, gently and appropriately move into action.

Some would argue that *any* action will help move us into healing because it creates movement among the stuckness and repetition. I have a lot of time for this idea and have witnessed the power of extremely simple daily changes repeated over months (making the bed, writing a gratitude list, showering every morning, walking round the block). These 'small' changes can interrupt old beliefs and patterns, so have a much bigger effect over time.

Although 'any action is good action' is probably true, it's too broad to be useful to everyone. How then do we know what action to take? How do we find a path up the mountain towards the sacred place?

The answer is that that we need to focus our action on developing the capacities that are currently limited or entirely missing because of our trauma and the patterns of dysregulation it has locked us into. As we heal, we develop many different, new capacities. For example, the capacity to pause, the capacity to allow our biological impulse (for example, we might notice that our body needs to stretch or shake and we allow it to do so), the capacity to separate from and see our wounding, the capacity to feel and then act on our embodied, instinctive, adult *no*.

These capacities and more develop over time as we heal our trauma. But the reverse is also true: actively working towards developing these capacities by taking appropriate daily action facilitates trauma healing. Viewed this way, it's clear that trauma healing is not an elusive, mystical thing, it's something we can all learn and master.

There are four overarching capacities that we need to develop and integrate so we can reach the mountain top. Over time, we need to develop the capacities to signal safety to our nervous system; to move into conscious awareness; to connect to our adult self; and to reclaim our agency. I explain these in detail on page 134. Learning and practising these capacities is the key to healing trauma. The joy of this capacity building approach is that the process is self-led: *you* can take action, every single day, to develop and strengthen each of them. This is, of course, the main message of this book. It's a call to action to help you unlock your power to heal yourself. But there's an important nuance to this message too, because although I want you to act, I also want you to ask for help when you need it.

Other people can help you learn, develop and integrate the capacities you need. At the right time, a Somatic Experiencing (SE) practitioner could help you feel safer in your body. A breathwork practitioner could help you increase your capacity for presence and conscious awareness. An Internal Family Systems (IFS) practitioner could help you develop a greater capacity to respond to every part of yourself with adult perspective and compassion. A coach could help you develop your capacity to take and maintain instinctive self-led action.

I want this book to empower you and light a spark in you. I want you to understand where you're currently at, the direction you need to head and what you need to do to get there. And as you feel your sense of power and agency rise, I want you to take appropriate, gentle action. But I don't want you to do it alone.

I had to take many steps as I found my way out of the forest and up the mountain, but I couldn't have done it without support and connection. One day at a time, I moved into agency and took action, but I was guided, loved (and at times cajoled) to where I needed to be. As you better understand what this whole weird trauma healing thing is about, you can choose when and how you want other people to help you make your way up the mountain.

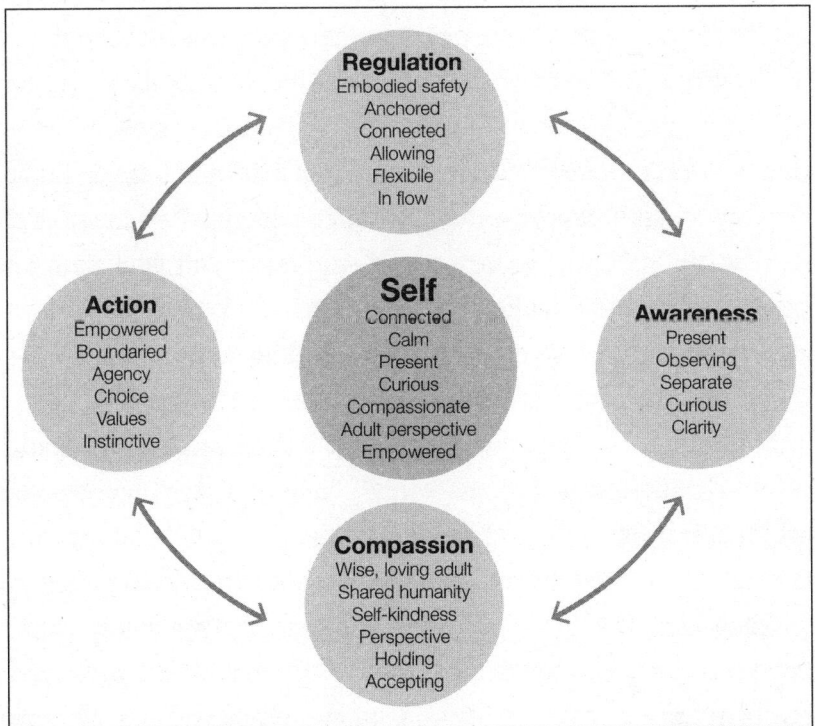

Diagram 3: The process of trauma healing

As we repeat this process – learning to feel safer in our body, regulating our nervous system, deepening our awareness and adult compassion, and empowering ourselves by recliming our agency and choice – we re-establish our sense of adult self and heal our trauma.

Trauma healing

As I've said earlier, all change starts with increased awareness – however, our awareness is facilitated by an increased sense of *safety*.

We must move into awareness slowly, in conjunction with an increased sense of safety in our bodies, or the awareness itself is traumatic and too much. Regulating our nervous systems and feeling safe powers the process of change and healing, allowing us to take meaningful, aligned action in a way that facilitates integration and reconnection with our adult self.

Diagram 3 illustrates the process of trauma healing. Before I describe each capacity in more detail, I want to make it clear that we don't move through this process just once. As we build nervous system capacity, move from contraction to release and regulation, become aware of and separate from our trauma, become compassionately able to 'be with' and tolerate the new awareness, move into empowerment and agency, and take new, different, expansive action, we create more embodied safety, and because of this, our awareness increases. We naturally move through this process, gently releasing tension, seeing and integrating more and more, and over time re-establish our connection to our true self and create a whole new way of being.

Each capacity positively affects and feeds into every other capacity. For example, as we build our capacity for presence, curiosity and conscious awareness, we naturally increase our capacity to signal safety to our nervous system. As we increase our capacity to receive ourselves with perspective and compassion, we increase our capacity for awareness. An increase in one capacity naturally leads to an increase in another, and vice versa.

Each evolution around the cycle creates a greater sense of embodied safety, widens our window of tolerance, interrupts old trauma-led patterns, integrates parts of ourselves, moves us from contraction to release, creates a solid sense of empowerment and agency, and re-establishes connection to our adult self. Trauma healing happens in a spiral as we move through this process. As each layer of the trauma and ourselves unfolds we go deeper, slowing moving towards the centre – the wounding.

Self-led action

Trauma healing is a slow process of moving from trauma-led action, where our wounding and survival adaptations subconsciously drive our actions, to self-led action, where our embodied, regulated, curious, compassionate, present, consciously aware adult self chooses how we act.

Agency refers to our sense of control and influence over ourselves and our life, and trauma has a detrimental impact on it. Subconsciously, we do not feel in control. Nor do we feel consistently able to take action that leads to a meaningful outcome. In part, this is because we're so stuck in the survival response and our old patterning. But it's also a deeper wounding, where part of us thinks we have little choice, that we cannot do things differently, that life is hard, and heartbreakingly, that we do not deserve to have a different experience of life.

Trauma is the outcome of feeling simultaneously threatened, overwhelmed and powerless. We were unable to act and respond, and it left us with a lingering sense of powerlessness. We subconsciously feel unable to create real change, and simply do not believe that healing, flow and connection are possible for us.

Many of us live with a subconscious sense that our bodies, lives and experience are out of our control. This can manifest as an overwhelming sense that we can't manage our lives, or as an urgent, clawing sense that we must control every detail of life. Often we swing between the two – moving from overwhelm and powerlessness into tight patterns of control.

Trauma subconsciously disconnects us from our innate agency and power. It also disconnects us from flow and a sense of possibility. Trauma healing, then, is about slowly reclaiming these natural states. We do this as we tentatively begin to interrupt the old patterns we're stuck in by beginning to take self-led action.

Increased capacity to take self-led action, rather than trauma-led action, is the outcome of increased nervous system regulation, conscious awareness, compassion and agency. *And* self-led action powers your journey through the process of trauma healing. This, really, is the central thesis of this book. Embodying safety requires you to take self-led action. Becoming aware requires you to take self-led action. Learning to reconnect to and respond from your adult self requires you to take self-led action. Unlocking your agency and power requires you to take, you guessed it, self-led action.

Some self-led action is visible and relational – it affects how we relate to the world and/or those around us. For example, it might look like turning down an invitation, a coffee or a dessert because you can feel that your nervous system needs down-regulation rather than stimulation. But more often self-led action is internal and not visible to others. For example, choosing to inhale twice and then exhale deeply while letting your muscles soften and ease, and repeating this as often as you need, is a simple act, imperceptible to others, that can increase your embodied sense of safety. Choosing to slow down and pause so you become aware of the tightness in your chest and a rising sense of anxiety is a self-led act that deepens your conscious awareness. Choosing to say to yourself, 'It's okay, I know you're afraid, this will pass' so you can *be with* the uncomfortable sensation is a self-led act that increases your capacity to tolerate and hold your discomfort. The result of choosing these actions is an increased sense of agency and power – and an increased capacity for more self-led action.

The most important word in these examples is *choosing.* Over time, as our nervous system becomes more flexible, as we increase our conscious awareness, and learn to operate from our wise, loving adult self, self-led action becomes our spontaneous default. But to get there we must actively *choose* self-led actions to reshape our inner and outer worlds.

As with every aspect of trauma healing, building our capacity to take self-led action is a slow process. We do this one day at time, making and sustaining small incremental changes. And as we do, we unlock our agency – slowly coming to see, feel and believe that we have control and influence over ourselves and our lives. As we reclaim our agency, we unlock our power to self-heal. We also begin to create the life we want.

Embodied safety

The biggest change in the trauma field over the past twenty years is our deepening understanding that trauma is primarily *about* the body. It's becoming laughable to think that we used to try and heal trauma only by talking about it because the more we know, the clearer it is that trauma exists in the body. The statement 'trauma exists in the body' doesn't mean that your traumatic experiences are eerily locked away in a weird little flesh-coloured bubble somewhere near your pancreas. What it means is that the traumatic reaction (i.e. fight-flight-freeze-fawn-collapse) is experienced first and foremost in the nervous system and the body. If we experience this reaction over and over again (as those with complex trauma and chronic patterns of dysregulation do) it affects our entire body. If you need some convincing on this, review page 97 for an overview of toxic stress and the body.

Those with childhood trauma have been living in survival mode physiologically. Driven by our neural survival maps and nervous system dysregulation, our bodies are contracted, tense and imbalanced. Because the tension and contraction (and the wounding that drives this contraction) is painful, we cope by disconnecting from our body. But the result of the disconnection (such as hiding in the mind, distracting ourselves, numbing out with alcohol) is more tension and contraction, because we don't interrupt, release or soothe the physiological survival response.

Trauma healing, then, is synonymous with helping our bodies move out of embodied survival and into embodied safety. But this isn't something that can be achieved quickly. There's no magic pill. And I mean this literally. Although certain medications, such as anti-depressants, or supplements such as magnesium, can help at the right time, they cannot take action to regulate your nervous system. You need to support this as, moment by moment, you practise and prioritise self-led action aimed at helping your beautiful body feel a little safer through soothing, anchoring, connecting and releasing.

Historically, within trauma treatment, helping a client feel safer has been a precursor – the initial stabilisation phase a clinical psychologist does before they get to the deep, meaningful work of, say, EMDR (Eye Movement Desensitisation and Reprocessing). We now know this perception is wildly incorrect. Regulating your nervous system is not the thing you do *before* you do your trauma healing. Regulating your nervous system *is* trauma healing. This new understanding is one of the main drivers that's tipping the balance of power in the field of trauma healing and mental health. Because although a practitioner, psychotherapist, psychiatrist or coach can help you co regulate during a session, the power to help your nervous system and signal safety to your body lies with you.

If you've spent your whole life feeling unsafe and disconnected from your body, what I've just said might feel unrealistic. Know you're not alone – most of my clients arrive with very little embodied experience of 'regulated and safe'. They, like you, don't know what the mountain top looks or feels like. Your lack of embodied experience of regulation and safety is normal in this world of trauma healing.

Feeling safer in your body is first and foremost about learning how to signal safety to your nervous system. There are many ways to do this, and I'll go into detail in Chapter Six. For now, and to keep it simple, it's helpful to think of this as taking action to help your body feel a little more at ease, by signalling comfort and safety in a conscious way. To do this, you need to begin to notice things that feel good to your body and do them more. These might be smiling, exhaling, stretching, being in nature, placing your hand on your heart, snuggling under a blanket, walking in the grass with your shoes off, laughing, cuddling someone, cuddling yourself, cuddling your pet, taking a warm shower or bath, or doing yoga, dance or *any* movement.

Triggered reactions and dysregulation disconnect us from the present moment, our body and other people. This disconnection aims to protect us, but in doing so leads to us feeling unsafe. Feeling safer is synonymous with gently reconnecting, and any of the actions I've just listed can potentially help us do that. They help us feel safer because we create a little more release and ease in our body while also anchoring back into the present moment instead of being lost in an old reaction.

Signalling safety also requires increased awareness of when we feel dysregulated, disconnected, unsafe and uncomfortable. Over time, we aim to become responsive and flexible – noticing when we're moving into survival and then taking action to regulate by signalling safety. As we do this, we build capacity in our nervous system, moving from rigid autopilot into responsive flow.

One of the first self-led acts I ask of my clients is for them to become deeply curious about how and when their body moves into fight-flight. I want them to begin to notice the contraction in their chest, a sense that things are speeding up, their heightened sense of alertness and their increased heart rate. I also want them to pay attention to their minds because, particularly for those of us who have spent our lives in our heads, noticing changes to our thinking can be easier. They might notice their thoughts racing, or catastrophic thinking. They might label these things 'anxiety', but we begin to call it what it is – the nervous system moving them into survival. Some clients feel like they skip fight-flight and jump straight to freeze, fawn or collapse. Likewise, I ask them to get curious about how their body moves into these states. As we clear the decks it becomes clear that fight-flight was happening, often many hours or days before, but because stress and tension feel normal – they're the baseline experience – they don't register the somatic changes.

The next self-led act, once they have developed a little more curiosity and capacity to notice the process of moving into survival, is to respond by signalling safety to their nervous system. We learn through trial and error what works for us and what doesn't. The self-led action we take when we're at the front end of fight-flight will be different to what we'll do when we're in collapse.

One of my clients, Rose, is a high-level emergency nurse. Her job is demanding and the stakes are high. As Rose became increasingly embodied, aware and compassionate, and as she anchored into her adult self, she became aware that she was moving intensely into fight-flight-freeze during emergency resuscitations. Her response is appropriate and completely understandable, but it was also preventing her from operating with clarity of thought, presence and confidence during these difficult moments at work. Over time, and through trial and error, she discovered that pausing before she stepped in, embodying (moving her attention down to her body), standing up tall and taking up space, exhaling and saying to herself, 'I am calm, I've got this' anchored her back into the present moment and signalled safety to her nervous system. Rose has experienced a very high level of trauma in her life, so her increased capacity to take self-led action in this way is remarkable, and illustrates what can be possible once you start.

Another client who experiences freeze as confusion, panic and overwhelm finds that putting her hand on her heart and slowing her breathing down (first in for two, out for two to balance her breath, then gradually moving to in for two, out for three, then in for two, out for four) brings her back. And another client who often experiences collapse as despair and a sensation that she's powering down (eyes closing, no muscle strength) finds that circling her hips while smiling (as if she's hula-hooping) brings her almost straight back into the present moment and out of collapse. I'm going to go into more detail about these tools in Chapter Six; now I'm just showing you some examples of how helping your body feel safer depends on a) which kind of survival response you're experiencing and b) your own physiology, preferences, likes and dislikes. The one thing all these clients did, and continue to do, is take self-led action.

I often say to clients, particularly those who are really stuck, that to begin with, 'we're going to have to *wrestle* your nervous system back into rhythm'. I hate using this language, but experience lets me know that it's 100 per cent true. Some are so deeply stuck in survival that curiously observing and compassionately responding in real time is impossible. For these clients we take it one day at a time, creating pockets of time in their day so they can deliberately self-regulate and release tension. In other words, rather than noticing and responding specifically to what's going on in their mind and body, I simply ask them to pause every hour and signal safety to their nervous system (whether they consciously think they need to or not!). This is how I moved out of collapse seven years ago – one sacred pause at a time.

Increased conscious awareness is the outcome of greater embodied safety and regulation. In other words, your capacity to see and feel yourself more clearly will deepen as you feel incrementally safer. Any self-led action you take to signal safety to your nervous system will quite naturally lead to an increased capacity to see, feel and 'hold' your trauma. As we make a little more space internally – as our muscles ease and release – our body and subconscious say, 'Ah, okay, here, you can know this now because *now* you can hold it.' This is a double-edged sword, because periods of glorious stabilisation and embodied safety are often followed by awareness of something old and painful. Knowing that what's happening is a positive sign of expansion and release and that you're being called to learn to hold, tolerate, see and love this old (new) pain is essential during these moments.

Awareness

Unresolved trauma, and all dysfunction, exists outside of conscious awareness. Unconscious patterning, denial, avoidance, disconnection and buried truths are the hallmark of families and individuals that are stuck and repeating old trauma-led patterns. Unresolved childhood trauma controls us because we cannot see it. Resolving trauma is about slowly, safely, and with support when necessary, moving our pain and patterning into conscious awareness. Gentle awareness, coupled with greater tolerance and acceptance, is trauma healing. Trauma healing, then, is a commitment to awareness – to seeing ourselves and our lives truthfully.

Conscious awareness creates a gap between you and your trauma-led patterns. Even if this gap is tiny – just a fleeting moment of observation, separation, seeing and knowing – it's a powerful first step as we move from being controlled by our trauma to being able to separate from it. This gap occurs as we pause and consciously step back, separating and learning to observe ourselves with a little more presence and perspective. This pause moves you out of autopilot, anchoring you back into the present moment and into self. For this reason, a pause is phenomenally powerful, as it interrupts our deeply embedded trauma-led patterning. It also moves us back into agency – as we pause, we become increasingly able to *choose* how we want to respond.

When we can separate even slightly from our triggered reaction, from our thinking, our emotions, our sensations, our behaviour, we are no longer *in it*. As you move through the process of trauma healing (creating more embodied safety, developing greater awareness, moving into more compassion and feeling a deeper sense of agency) the gap between you and your trauma widens, and your connection to self as a presence and observer feels robust, reliable and solid.

We move into conscious awareness and reconnect to self when we:

- Pause
- Become present (moving into our senses and/or our body)
- Observe ourselves with a little more distance and perspective
- Move into curiosity.

Over time, as we increasingly observe and separate from a place of greater embodied safety, compassion and agency, we slowly become aware of:

- The triggers in the environment and in our thinking, emotions and body that pull us into the survival response
- How we experience each aspect of the survival response (fight, flight, freeze, fawn and collapse)
- How, when and why we disconnect from our adult self, our body and the world
- Our survival adaptations: the behavioural, emotional and cognitive survival strategies and protective parts of our personalities we developed to cope/avoid the wounding
- Our wounding: the unseen wounded parts of ourselves, old emotions, sensations, thoughts and traumatic beliefs.

As the layers unfold and we integrate, embody and anchor into our adult self we also become aware of:

- Our emotions and sensations
- Embodied comfort, goodness and hope
- More flow and flexibility
- Our agency, power and right to choose

- Our instinct and intuition
- Our body's natural rhythm
- Our boundaries and limits
- Our needs and wants
- Our increased capacity
- Our natural desire to connect to safe people and the world.

Moving into awareness – separating from and curiously observing something related to our trauma – is often triggering. Moving what was unconscious into conscious awareness is a wild ride because the things we're trying to see, hold and move towards often feel too much. We often find ourselves moving between increased curiosity and awareness and then into survival, overwhelm, denial or resistance. First we might have a momentary realisation that feels something like this: 'I think I'm trying to control everyone and everything around me because I'm terrified of losing control, getting it all wrong and the worst happening to those I love.' Then, because the realisation feels too much, we either:

1. Dissociate.
2. Anxiously google 'how to stop being a control freak'.
3. Tidy the house . . . then the garden shed . . . then the car (while mentally repeating 'I'm not a control freak').
4. Eat a packet of salty nuts at breakneck speed.
5. Feel an intense rage at that idiot Sarah Woodhouse who wrote that stupid fucking book that made you 'curiously observe' all this shit that was better left in the box collecting dust.

There are a great many other response options too – I just picked my own personal favourites. My point is that because the awareness itself is triggering, we must prioritise increasing our embodied sense of safety, and our capacity to tolerate and *hold* our new awareness. If we don't do this, the awareness feels too much, so we simply get pulled back into disconnection and survival.

Awareness itself is a skill, a core capacity, that we learn, practise and nurture. We practise slowing down, pausing, getting curious about what's going on. We practise observing ourselves, slowly becoming willing to see ourselves – and reality – with increased clarity. We go from moving head down, in autopilot, unconsciously unwilling to do things differently, to pausing, getting curious and interested in ourselves and our reactions, and inviting *reality* to show itself. Slowly we become able to be present with, and aware of, things that previously felt too much.

Compassion

Polyvagal Theory has taught us that when we're regulated and feeling safe, we naturally and more easily connect to compassion. The reverse is also true. When we're dysregulated and in survival we struggle to connect to this essential human trait. This is highly problematic for those of us stuck in survival. Instead of responding to ourselves, our weakness, our fears and our mistakes from a regulated, embodied state of gentle compassion, we respond from our wounding and our survival adaptations.

Often in place of internal compassion is shaming, fear, criticism, catastrophising, self-blame and self-hate. How we respond reflects our survival state, but it also reflects how we were received in childhood. As children, when our mistakes, our weakness or our fears are received with presence, regulation and kindness, we learn to do the same. If, however, we were not consistently received in this way, we internalise whatever response we were met with.

Receiving ourselves with compassion is a capacity in and of itself – something to gently practise and explore as you walk this path. Before I explain more about this capacity, I need to tell you something that might sting. The fact is: trauma healing isn't possible without increased self-compassion. Developing this capacity is essential, not optional. I dearly wish someone had been this straightforward with me. I saw therapists who received me with compassion and highlighted to me when I was being ferociously unkind to myself. But they never said: 'The capacity to meet yourself with increased compassion and be the wise, loving adult you need is the foundation of trauma healing – develop this capacity and you will heal; avoid this and you won't.'

That was what I needed to hear. I needed someone to highlight that compassion isn't just a lovely, fluffy optional extra. I needed someone to tell me that becoming able to *parent* myself was the only option I had if I wanted to be well, to thrive and to grow.

Why do some therapists and psychologists fear using this kind of language? Why do we resist telling our clients, at the right time, precisely what they're aiming for? I think about this a lot and I'm concerned. I'm concerned because *not* telling a client where they need to aim and how they can help themselves get there disempowers them. *Not* telling a client leaves the therapist with all the power – watching and waiting for silent shifts in the client as they slowly move through a passive process. I'm not suggesting therapists do this deliberately, but nonetheless I believe subconscious disempowerment is often the outcome of such a hands-off approach to trauma healing.

I have gently told clients this truth and held space for the painful reaction that has unfolded in response. I have been present with their anger, their grief, their sadness and their overwhelming sense that it is not fair. Again, I need to emphasise: *Yes, it is not fair.* It is not fair that you were not consistently met with compassion, presence and reason as a child. It is not fair that you need to learn to do this. It is not fair that no-one else can do it for you. It is not fair, but it is true. Shying away from this truth will not help you heal. Gently moving towards this truth, while being aware of your reaction and then helping your body feel safer after this reaction, is the only way to the other side. *This* is trauma healing. And as you do this, you will widen your window of tolerance, move into acceptance and, ironically, build your capacity to receive yourself with compassion.

Here, I want to draw your attention to the work of psychologist Kristin Neff, the queen of compassion. She researches it and creates powerful interventions and tools designed to help us all create more of it. Neff asserts that there are three main elements of compassion: mindfulness, common humanity and self-kindness.

Mindfulness

Neff tells us that self-compassion requires taking a balanced, mindful approach to our suffering so that we neither suppress nor exaggerate it. Mindfulness is, of course, simply another way of understanding conscious awareness. Both Neff and I are moving you in the same direction – connection to the present moment and the capacity to separate from and observe your trauma in a different way. Neff includes conscious awareness in her definition of compassion, which highlights the inter-twined, connected nature of awareness and compassion. Neff writes: 'Mindfulness allows us to turn toward our pain with acceptance of the present moment reality. It prevents us from becoming *over-identified* with difficult thoughts and feelings, so we aren't swept away by negative reactivity.'[3] Amen to that. One of the primary purposes of increased awareness is that it creates space, and a gap between *us* and our pain. Neff asserts that as we move into 'self as observer', we naturally move towards compassion.

Common humanity

Self-compassion involves being able to recognise that all humans suffer. Neff writes: 'the very definition of being human means being vulnerable, flawed and imperfect. When we are self-compassionate, we recognise that our suffering connects us rather than separates us from others.'[4] This second aspect of compassion is all about connection and perspective. In our trauma we become so singular – thinking we are the only one who has trauma, the only one who is triggered, the only one who is struggling. 'I am failing, but everyone else is thriving' is a common active belief for those with trauma. Where someone without trauma may experience anxiety and internally respond with a deep sense that anxiety is a shared human experience, those with childhood trauma feel as if the anxiety itself is a sign of their failure and aloneness. To move into compassion, we practise responding to ourselves in a way that reconnects us back to humanity. For example, saying to ourselves, 'everyone is triggered sometimes' is a simple but powerful way to 'right-size' the problem we face, anchor us to our adult perspective and self, and reconnect us back to our shared humanity.

Self-kindness

Self-compassion means being kind and understanding towards ourselves if we suffer, fail or feel inadequate, rather than ignoring our pain or self-flagellating with criticism. This inner support increases our embodied sense of safety and reconnects us to our sense of agency. Self-kindness is the most well-known aspect of compassion, but it's still worth taking a minute to consider what a kind and understanding response might sound like. One of the simplest ways to show ourselves kindness and understanding is by seeing and validating our experience. For example, saying to yourself, 'You're really over-whelmed right now – I get it, this morning has been stressful' is a powerful way to exercise self-kindness.

I love Neff's definition, because breaking it down this way makes the whole thing more approachable and less 'just love yourself'. The term self-compassion is so entwined with a saccharine version of self-kindness that we can struggle to see that it's a much more grounded, adult, solid *thing* than simply showering ourselves in affirmations.

Self-compassion *is* adulting. It's about reconnecting to our grounded, wise adult self so we can move into trauma healing and create real change in ourselves and in our lives.

Chapter Five

The self-led approach

The self-led approach to trauma healing is designed to empower you to create a new way of living that heals your trauma. More than anything, I want you to understand that *you* hold the power to heal yourself. As intoxicating and delicious as this statement is, it's also true that to access this power you need to learn *how*. We can't simply flick a switch and start healing – we need to practise and develop this new way of being and relating.

This chapter is your how-to guide to integrating the four core capacities so you can find your way to the mountain top. We won't focus on the detail of what to do day-to-day – that will come in Chapters Six, Seven, Eight and Nine – but rather on explaining the overarching Principles of Self-led Integration in more detail.

Self-led integration

My approach is officially called Self-led Integration™. I've chosen to use the word *integration* instead of *healing* because 'integration' tells you something very important about what you're aiming for.

Integration is the process of bringing separate pieces together to form a unified whole. Over time, as we move through trauma healing, we integrate (consolidate, assimilate and *own*) different capacities by learning and practising them. We also integrate the parts of ourselves that we've pushed away into our adult self – seeing our wounding and accepting ourselves as we truly are. Integrating these new capacities and our authentic self leads to a new sense of wholeness. *Integration* is the process of trauma healing. *Integrated* is the mountain top. As we make our way up the mountain we integrate:

- The four core capacities of trauma healing
- The Principles of Self-led Integration
- The parts of ourselves we've pushed away
- Our wisest adult self
- Past memories, emotions and perspectives.

As we integrate the four core capacities of trauma healing, the principles and our sense of self, we create a deep, reassuring sense of wholeness. It might sound complex, but in reality we integrate quite simply, through daily action and repetition, and by sticking to some overarching trauma healing principles.

Neuroplasticity: The pros

The powering force behind the process of integration is neuroplasticity – as I mentioned on page 93, this is the nervous system's ability to change itself constantly by creating new neural pathways and losing those which are no longer used. Our actions, thoughts, environment, emotions, body and nervous system all interact constantly, and what we think, do and then repeat directly affects how our nervous system is wired. Behaviours, actions and thoughts that we repeat often are supported by strong neural pathways. Repeated actions become automatic, habitual and unconscious, so we don't have to think or focus to do them. They become *integrated* into our being. Think of how you press the brake of a car when you need to stop without focusing or thinking about it. But when you were learning to drive, you had to focus very hard on this action because it wasn't embedded – you did not have a neural imprint of it. This skill hadn't been fully integrated, but because you repeated the action, it became automatic over time.

An action becomes subconscious and automatic thanks to neuroplasticity, which, as I previously explained, is to blame for our deeply embedded, automatic trauma responses. But the good news is that it's also the self-led power that will move you out of autopilot and into deep healing and real change.

Research shows that it takes between 18 to 254 days to make a new action an unconscious habit, with an average of 66 days.[1] In the study, the length of time it took to integrate a new action depended on the type of new habit the participant was trying to embed. Simple actions, like drinking a glass of water every day, became automatic more quickly than more difficult ones like daily exercise. As blindingly obvious as this conclusion is, I think it's reassuring to know that even if the action is complex, *doing it differently* will become our new normal if we commit to the unsexy but extremely powerful concept of daily self-led action and repetition.

The four capacities

Learning and practising the four capacities of trauma healing constitutes doing it *differently*. These capacities are:

- Capacity One: Signalling safety to your nervous system and self-regulating.
- Capacity Two: Moving into presence, observation, curiosity and clarity.
- Capacity Three: Receiving yourself with perspective and compassion.
- Capacity Four: Unlocking your agency and taking self-led action.

These capacities involve learning and practising many others along the way. For example, our capacity to regulate our nervous system is bound up with the ability to be in our body, increasingly experiencing life anchored in our physicality; being able to tolerate feelings and sensations, noticing and 'being with' uncomfortable ones; and being able to sense how the body wants to move and allowing it. The four capacities I've listed are not the whole picture, but they give necessary direction and structure to the action we take every day.

The following four chapters look at one capacity at a time. As you use the tools and techniques outlined in each chapter, you'll integrate these new ways of being. Each capacity, together with the principles that accompany them, harnesses and unlocks the power of neuroplasticity. As you practise, you will move yourself and your nervous system into the learning zone and begin to create real change at a neural level. Over time, the self-led action changes your brain, moving you into agency and self-efficacy – out of autopilot, to a place where you can reclaim your right to choose how you show up in life.

Before we get started, though, I need to pause and make an important point – maybe the most important point in the book. In Chapter Three: The consequences, I explained that people often know a lot about trauma healing but struggle to actually put it into practice. I say this without judgement and with a huge amount of solidarity and compassion. This was me before my diagnosis – knowing a lot, talking a lot, but not taking daily action to create a new way of living. I, like these clients, was in freeze – frozen by the possibility of making a mistake. As you move into the next four chapters, remember this. If you read them but don't gently move into action, nothing will shift. It's the action that will heal you.

Compassionate consistency

To get a sense of how other practitioners encourage their clients to establish new habits, I spoke to Dane Ensley, the warm, engaging CEO and founder of Reconstruction Unlimited (RU), a mental health consultancy based in LA and London. RU creates bespoke teams of coaches, practitioners, psycho-therapists and psychiatrists around their clients. When I say *around* their clients, I mean this literally. Some of their coaches even live with the client, making sure that from morning to night the client is moving in the right direction. Taking a peek into how they do what they do is fascinating and gives us deep insight into how to create real, long-lasting change. As Dane explained:

I think as sensitive humans and as a sensitive culture, we're collectively uncomfortable promoting the importance of personal discipline. Discipline feels like such a harsh word, particularly in the trauma space. But consistency is essential if we want to create real change. Repeating specific actions moves you in the direction you need to go. This isn't necessarily the direction that you *want* to go in, but it's the direction that your wisest self knows that you *need* to go in. We don't always want to act. But you can't sit around and wait to get enlightened. You have to walk up the hill. And you don't just do it once, you do it over and over and over and over and over again.

Admiral McRaven said: 'If you want to change the world, start by making your bed every morning.' And it's true! My life changed because I was taught to make my bed as an adult. I started making my bed and I never stopped making my bed. The bed gets made no matter what. This action was small enough for me to find 100 per cent consistency around it. But it was also different enough to create ripples in my life and break patterns. Making the bed demonstrated a new commitment to self-respect. To this day it signals to me the type of man I want to be as I approach the day.

Dane continued:

My life is always changing, so I need concrete actions and habits to anchor me. Making my bed is one of these anchors. So is my morning routine. I meditate then I read a short spiritual text, then I grab my notebook and write for three minutes. I've done this pretty much every day for fifteen years. The familiarity is soothing. Just like making my bed, the morning routine reminds me that I'm choosing to live my live in a disciplined, honest way. Everyone needs their own version of this morning routine. It doesn't matter what the routine consists of. What matters is the consistency and the repetition – this is the anchor and the act that can change the course of your whole day.

When Dane and his team parachute into someone's life, they focus first on re-establishing discipline through repetition. They create daily anchors for their clients – anchors that interrupt old patterns and reconnect people to their adult self. They do this because they understand that repetition is the only way to create long-lasting change at a neural level. Remember the analogy of making the bed, or Dane's simple morning routine, as you move into self-led action. It's not about creating radical changes to your day-to-day life. It's about creating a change you can commit to and finding consistency with it.

To help you do this, make the action smaller than you think you need it to be. For example, if you're aiming to develop Capacity Two (being present, curious and consciously aware) through meditation, don't set yourself the goal of meditating for fifteen minutes twice a day. Instead, set yourself the goal of meditating once a day for two minutes. Once you can repeat this action consistently, increase it. Build change slowly, repeating small, achievable actions that will help you integrate the four core capacities, and you will create deep, meaningful, long-lasting change that's supported at a neural level.

By the way, I can already hear you berating yourself for missing a day, so I'll add a suggestion here. Instead of using the concepts of consistency, discipline and daily anchors to beat yourself up, shall we use them in a new way? Allow yourself to practise and fail, as all humans do. Allow yourself to be compassionate in your approach. You do not have to do this perfectly. You do not have to hold yourself to the same standard as Admiral McRaven, or Dane for that matter.

One of my favourite facts, which I repeat endlessly to my children whenever they make a mistake, is that optimal learning requires us to fail about 15 per cent of the time.[2] If we never fail, we're not learning. Potentially we're either aiming too low (learning something at a lower level than we're actually capable) or we're pushing ourselves too hard (so we're too stressed to learn). Likewise, if we fail more than about 15 per cent of the time, we're either aiming too high or there's something else going on.

Fifteen per cent failure is not just human – it's ideal if we want to learn. I'm happy to report that I think I've probably failed at about 15 per cent of this day. I frequently move out of consistency. I miss things. I forget things I've committed to. Sometimes I make my bed at 8 pm, just before I get into it (which on reflection is a little weird). Here's the difference between me today and the me of twenty years ago: today when I fail, I smile. I hold my humanness with adult perspective and compassion. Just like building the habit of making my bed, I had to learn and practise compassionately responding to myself when I forgot to do it. Twenty years ago, I could not access my own adult compassion, perspective or wisdom. I could not be the wise, loving adult that I so desperately needed. I had to learn this and practise it through daily self-led action. Over time I integrated this capacity – I made it my own. Automatically responding with compassion and perspective has replaced automatically responding with self-hate and panic. Just as I learned this, so can you.

Not making my bed, making it at 8 pm, or forgetting any of the other multitude of things I 'should' do now simply prove to me that I'm human. No longer do I receive my humanness as proof that I'm defective or a failure. I receive myself with compassion because I know that responding with a lack of compassion will pull me back into old patterns of shame and low self-worth that no longer serve me. Neuroplasticity is harnessed through repetition and consistency, but it's also contingent on self-compassion, which keeps us regulated and connected to our adult self. Compassionate consistency, then, is the only way to approach self-led integration because it ensures we widen our window of tolerance rather than being pulled back into trauma-led patterns of self-blame.

This is going to hurt

As part of the research for this book I also spoke to Ingrid Clayton, a clinical psychologist based in Los Angeles. She specialises in trauma, using EMDR, Somatic Experiencing and an Internal Family Systems (IFS) framework to help her clients find their way up the mountain. Ingrid is disarmingly funny, silly and sweary. She also has a trauma history, which I suspect explains the 'funny, silly, sweary' part of her personality. So many who have been dealt brutal blows by life come out the other side with a darkly beautiful sense of humour and are quick to laugh. It makes sense. 'Gallows humour' is a pretty smart survival adaptation. Ingrid and I talked for a long time, and so much of what she shared about her fifteen years in practice and her own healing journey was extremely powerful. But it's one of the first things she said to me that I feel called to share with you here. I asked Ingrid to explain to me how she helps a client start this work. Here's what she said:

The first thing I do is tell a client that they're going to feel unsafe. We so often make trauma healing and self-care sound like it'll feel like a victory lap, but taking care of ourselves does not feel good. It actually feels terrifying, scary, exhausting and overwhelming. Even when we know the stakes aren't that high. For example, say you need to talk to your landlord because your air conditioning isn't working. But oh my God, you cannot have the conversation. It makes sense that it's so hard, because you're going against the thing that's always kept you safe – avoiding conflict, keeping the peace, fawning and people-pleasing, say.

So I ask my client: can we just be present to that? Just put your hand on your heart, skin to skin like when a baby is born so we're releasing oxytocin, and say to yourself, 'I am here and this is hard.'

Because we're not supposed to transcend the difficulty of it. This is the work. The work is *being with* the difficulty of it. It sucks and it's hard, and it might bring up a lot of grief and tears, and maybe you can't speak to your landlord today, but today you can notice how hard it is – and the awareness is amazing. The pacing, the presence and being in compassionate relationship to self, I think are the building blocks of regulation and safety.

This is going to hurt is, essentially, the first thing Ingrid tells a client. I'm telling you here, before you move into self-led action, because the reality of this work needs to be made clear. Building your capacity to tolerate what is currently intolerable is not a comfortable, easy task. It, quite literally, requires you to do things that currently feel uncomfortable. The *uncomfortable things* are all designed to help you grow in the direction you want to grow. They're self-led and aligned. They're not random acts of self-flagellation. They serve a purpose because they interrupt old trauma-led patterns and move you up the mountain. The action we take is personal and contingent on where we're at. For one person, the uncomfortable thing that will help them grow and widen their window of tolerance might be speaking to their landlord. For another, it could be holding eye contact with their partner.

All my clients practise different uncomfortable things based on where they're at and the direction they want to go. One client is practising tolerating driving her car on a motorway; another is currently practising consistent self-care by showering daily and eating at the table instead of hovering by the fridge. Each action is equally uncomfortable for them. But they aren't simply pushing through the pain, they're learning to support themselves through the discomfort.

This is going to hurt is true of trauma healing. But it's not a masochistic exercise. We learn to tolerate small amounts of discomfort; we do not force ourselves into actions that will trigger and harm us. Slow and steady, stretching ourselves without stressing ourselves is how we integrate and create real change.

Building tolerance

Window of tolerance is a term coined by Dr Dan Siegel. It refers to the zone we can operate in without getting stressed or overwhelmed. Those with unresolved trauma have a narrow window of tolerance, meaning that we can tolerate very little stress and stimulation in daily life. When we're in our window of tolerance, our ventral vagal nerve is active – we're present and connected. When we're pushed outside our window of tolerance we move into survival mode, and our unresolved trauma means we spend more time outside the window than inside it. Widening our window of tolerance is essential so we're not constantly in survival mode. Like everything I'm presenting here, it can be achieved outside of the clinic room through intentional self-led action in daily life.

The word 'tolerate' can sound inhospitable, as if I'm suggesting you learn simply to endure unpleasant feelings, but building our capacity to tolerate new uncomfortable actions, situations, sensations, emotions and realisations has nothing to do with endurance. In fact, it's the opposite. We develop the skill of noticing and being with discomfort (such as sensations of anxiety, grief or shame) for a short moment, and then take action to create more safety and comfort. Instead of staying stuck and locked into an overwhelming feeling or state, we first notice the discomfort, and then we consciously help ourselves feel safer/better. To use Peter Levine's terminology, we 'pendulate', gently flowing between discomfort and comfort. This allows us to experience our feelings in a safe way – to feel the safety that newly exists alongside the fear. As we learn and practise different tools designed to help us become increasingly comfortable with what was previously uncomfortable, we regulate our nervous system and widen our window of tolerance.

You can start playing with this idea now. As you move through your day, pause when you notice that you're anxious, worried, afraid, tense and so on. Name it as simply as you can (saying something like 'I'm feeling really anxious right now'). Move your attention to the part of your body that holds the anxious sensations. This gets you out of your mind and the story it's telling you about why you're experiencing the feeling, and into the feeling itself. Name what you feel using simple, clear language (for example, 'I experience this as tightness in my chest and jaw') and respond with compassion to bring a little more safety (such as saying, 'it's okay, everyone feels anxious sometimes, this will pass'). Next, allow the anxiety to be present, while keeping your attention on it – be with the sensations as they move. When you feel you've had enough, when the movement stops, or if it feels too much, move your attention away from the anxiety and use a tool to signal safety. For example, use the double-bump breath I describe on page 185 and then shake your body and jump on the spot. This process sometimes only takes twenty seconds, but it's a powerful way to begin to increase your tolerance by being with the anxious survival energy while feeling the presence of safety and containment alongside it.

The next chapter is all about Capacity One, and in it I describe loads of actions you can take to help your body feel more comfortable once you notice you're feeling discomfort. This movement into safety interrupts the survival response and (when repeated) widens our window of tolerance.

Sam, a lovely client of mine, dissociated intensely whenever the topic of his son's mental health came up in our sessions. It was highly triggering for Sam, making him instantly feel out of control, powerless and unsafe because it reminded him of his own childhood struggles. When the issue came anywhere near Sam's conscious awareness he was triggered. He couldn't *tolerate* the awareness, or the emotions that accompanied the awareness, which meant he could not move into self-led action and support his son in the way he wanted to. Very slowly, Sam practised first noticing how the triggered reaction manifested, and then took action, using soothing and anchoring techniques (see page 189) to help create more regulation and embodied safety. Slowly, and thanks to the action Sam took between our sessions, he became able to tolerate the awareness that his son was struggling. He did this by supporting himself and leaning into self-regulation and self-compassion. Approximately four months later, Sam came to the session saying, 'I need to talk about my son – he's not okay and I want to get him some help.' During our conversation, Sam used many tools to help himself remain in his body – taking gentle self-led action to signal safety to his nervous system. As a result, he was able to remain connected to his adult self during the conversation and then move into aligned, self-led action to help his son in the real world.

Sam's story illustrates that although we cannot rush this process of neural rewiring, if we take daily action to build capacity and widen our window of tolerance, we will see powerful, important changes emerge over time. We will become the adult we want to be.

Is this too much?

As well as noticing emotional discomfort in the body and supporting ourselves through it, we also need to become able to discern when something is simply too much for us. As you practise and integrate this idea you'll begin to understand when to 'hold yourself through the discomfort' and when something is simply too much for your nervous system.

This idea is so important to the self-led approach that it's one of the lead principles: stretch don't stress. This principle comes directly from Polyvagal Theory, as Stephen Porges and Deb Dana remind us that 'our goal in shaping new patterns is to stretch but not stress our nervous system. We want to stretch, feel the shape of a new pattern, and spend a moment savoring it. When we feel we need to power through an experience or suffer to see results, we stress the system and move into one of the survival states. Once that happens, we're no longer shaping. Instead, we're held in a familiar pattern of protection.'

In other words, growth requires you to stretch yourself gently to interrupt patterns and do things differently. But it also requires you to get an embodied sense of when something is too big, too triggering and too much for your system. Moving into trauma healing requires us to experience moments of manageable discomfort in our mind, emotions, relationships and body, but also to become our own protector – to say no, or simply stop, when an experience is too much for us.

The line of 'too much' differs day to day and moment to moment. When our capacity is higher – say we're well rested and feeling hopeful – our 'this is too much' line will be higher. We can tolerate more. When we're low capacity, our tolerance will be lower and smaller things can suddenly feel overwhelming and require us to move into endurance to get through. It's obvious, really: growth requires us to stretch ourselves, but not so much that we move back into survival. However, as obvious as this may seem intellectually, most people struggle to put this principle into practice. Trauma-led patterns are the main cause here. Because trauma disconnects us from our body, over time we lose touch with our capacity to tell when something is too much. Trauma healing reconnects us to our body, which in turn enables us to feel where our line of 'too much' is. The reverse is also true – as we set the intention of discovering and living by this line, we reconnect to our body and reinstate our boundaries.

Bea is a 36-year-old mother of three. We've been working together for about twelve months, and she's practising a lot of uncomfortable new self-led behaviours when she's with her mother, father and siblings. Previously, her pattern has been to disregard her own needs and boundaries and focus on pleasing others as a way of staying safe with her family of origin. Now, Bea tries to move slowly and mindfully despite her family's frantic, chaotic energy. She states her preferences and says 'no thank you' firmly when her overbearing, controlling mother tells her what to eat or where to sit. She tries to notice, and not act on, her need to fix and fawn if her father seems displeased or critical of her or her children. During these new behaviours Bea signals safety to her body (Capacity One), curiously observes herself and her emotions (Capacity Two) and internally speaks to herself with perspective and compassion (Capacity Three). Slowly, Bea is interrupting the old patterns and creating new ones.

But there are times when this is just too much for Bea. During highly stressful or emotional times in life, the most loving choice for Bea and her nervous system is to stay away from her family.

Julia Samuel is a psychotherapist and author, specialising in grief and loss. As we discussed the idea of knowing when not to push, Julia said:

There are times in life, maybe if we're experiencing loss or crisis, that we need to go back to basics. We cannot expect ourselves to push, to elevate or even, sometimes, to get out of bed.

Developing an embodied understanding of when something is too much for us is critical for healing. We must give ourselves permission to say 'no' to something, even if this something seems trivial, like popping to the shops or answering a phone call.

To heal we must replace 'shoulds', with a real sense of where our limits are.

Slowly, as we integrate the four capacities and follow the principles (which I explain on page 156), we find that our line of 'too much' (e.g. our window of tolerance) becomes higher and higher. But this will only come to pass if you also give yourself permission to acknowledge when something is too much.

A soft place to land

The self-led approach is about intentionally choosing a direction we want to go in and taking action that can feel uncomfortable. It's about taking personal responsibility for ourselves and our lives. It's the therapeutic equivalent of standing up and shouting: 'This is my life and I want it back.'

For this reason, as we move into self-led action, we need soft places to land. In other words, we need support. This could be a therapist, practitioner or psychologist. But it doesn't *have* to be. As Sat Dharam Kaur said:

We all need a cushion. That's what everybody needs – a place to feel safe and supported no matter what happens. It doesn't have to be a therapist. It could be a spiritual teacher. It could be a good friend. It could be a sibling, it could be a community member, it could be a priest. It just has to be someone non-judgmental who is going to listen.

In modern Western society it's hard to find people who can be our safe place to land. It's particularly hard if we've spent the past twenty years stuck in trauma-led patterns and on autopilot. So try to approach this idea gently, curiously and creatively.

A friend of mine is currently going through a divorce. She doesn't want or need to see a psychotherapist, but she understands that she needs a soft place to land as she takes action and creates change, so she's chosen to see a local reiki practitioner every week. As my lovely friend courageously implements changes in her life, this reiki practitioner provides an important space for authenticity, connection and letting go. Support matters, but it doesn't have to look how we're told it has to look. Finding people who feel safe, and where the connection feels gentle and non-judgemental, is often more important than qualifications.

Because trauma goes hand in hand with compulsive behaviours designed to help us cope, I often steer clients towards 12-step support groups. The 12-step fellowships started with Alcoholics Anonymous (AA) and there are now groups designed to help with pretty much any compulsive behaviour (such as compulsive eating, screen use, worrying, overworking, underearning, people-pleasing and so on).

The 12-step approach is about taking daily action while simultaneously moving into connection with something greater than ourselves. Everyone defines their own 'something greater' differently. Although for some it's a traditional concept of God, for many others it's a more nuanced concept of universal energy, presence or peace. What I've noticed in myself and my clients is that we naturally begin to experience a sense of connection to 'something greater than ourselves' as we integrate the four core capacities of trauma healing. This makes sense once we understand that trauma has had us locked into patterns of disconnection. In so many ways we've been disconnecting from the world around us – from awe and wonder, from presence and peace, from safety and grounding. Reconnecting back to these things (that are, by definition, 'something greater than ourselves') is what trauma healing is all about. In so many ways, then, the 12-step approach – with its emphasis on daily action and reconnection – is aligned with trauma healing.

Because many people associate the 12-step approach with extreme alcohol addiction and/or with an old-fashioned patriarchal religiosity, many who would benefit from this structured community solution dismiss, judge and avoid it. As you read this, try to notice if part of you reacts defensively. I want you to feel, state and act on your embodied 'no'. But it's also true that your trauma doesn't want you to change. Your trauma wants you to remain disconnected and repeating the same patterns. Something that, from the outside looking in, appears as radical and different as the 12-step approach is likely to elicit a strong, protective, fixed internal reaction. This is often a sign we've moved into survival, and that we're reacting rather than responding. The opposite of this protective reaction is regulation, curiosity and openness. Perhaps you can reach for a little more of this now by exhaling deeply, dropping your shoulders and relaxing your body. It's feasible that the 12-step approach will not be right for you, but you'll only be able to connect to your instinct and truth around this as you create a little more regulation and calm in your system. If you make this decision from survival, it's likely to be a trauma-led *reaction*, not a self-led *action*. You do not need to decide today whether you will or will not explore the 12-step approach. If you can, try and sit in the 'maybe'. Not knowing feels uncomfortable, but it will allow you to flow and find what you need, rather than reacting on autopilot.

From time to time clients need to attend Alcoholics Anonymous (AA), Cocaine Anonymous (CA), Overeaters Anonymous (OA) or Eating Disorders Anonymous (EDA). But more commonly I steer clients towards either Workaholics Anonymous (WA) or Adult Children of Alcoholics & Dysfunctional Families (ACA). WA is for those stuck in compulsive thinking, worrying, doing, activity and/or working. ACA is for those who often find themselves operating from a young, wounded place and feel somehow stuck as an 'adult child'.

Although initially the prospect of going to one of these online groups is terrifying, over time (as we become able to tolerate the discomfort) these groups of like-minded people, all focused on healing and growing, can become soft places to land. Some clients simply attend the meetings to listen and absorb. Some find a sponsor and work through the twelve steps. Others build up a robust support network over time, making connections that eventually become friendships. Either way, these groups provide an important, free support network for those committed to self-led action and breaking trauma-led patterns.

The 12-step groups are not perfect, but they're a good enough source of support for many. Whether you do or do not choose to explore the 12-step approach, trauma healing is hard, so do what you can to find soft places to land as you move through this work.

How to create a program

The next four chapters are a carefully constructed toolbox full of information, tools and techniques about integrating the four capacities. Before you continue reading, I want to steer you on how to use the rest of this book to create your own self-led program. I recommend reading to the end of this chapter and before you do anything else, spend a week playing with the principles (page 156). Familiarising yourself with these before you dive into the capacities will serve you well. Head to my website for a downloadable version of the principles – consider printing it out and sticking it somewhere you're going to see it.

Option one: Starting at the start
Move through Chapter Six (which covers the first capacity) slowly, implementing the tools and techniques you feel drawn to. Take notes and journal about your experience as you go to help you process and integrate. When you've completed Chapter Six, move onto the next capacity. Read and slowly implement each capacity in order. When you've completed Chapter Nine, read Chapter Ten to conclude what you've learned.

Option two: Start where you are
Once you've read and practised the principles described on page 156, head to the capacity you feel resonates the most (the one you're drawn to, intrigued by, or sense you need right

151

now). Slowly work through it, using the tools and techniques it outlines. Take notes and journal about your experience as you go. Take your time as you do this. When you're done, move on to the next capacity you feel drawn to. Or, if developing one capacity feels enough for now, read Chapter Ten to create a sense of conclusion. Use the principles and the capacity tools as the basis for your new way of living. Come back to the other capacity chapters at a later date, or just move on and trust you have taken in all you need for now.

There are pros and cons to both options – there's no perfect option that suits everyone. This need to find our own way and trust our choice can be very painful for those with trauma. Try to notice if this choice triggers anxiety, fear, worry, or paralysis.

The self-led approach is designed to build a new kind of anchored, regulated self-trust. Just as with all aspects of these capacities, we build this one moment at a time. Self-trust sounds lovely, but in reality involves a lot of emotional and cognitive discomfort. It's okay that it's uncomfortable – noticing the discomfort and responding differently will help us move out of autopilot. Noticing the discomfort that comes with making a choice and holding yourself through it, signalling safety to your nervous system and responding with self-compassion, is how we respond differently.

If you're unsure, allow yourself to be unsure! This is okay! Allow it and own it, saying something like, 'I'm unsure which option is going to work best for me and this feels uncomfortable' to yourself. This too builds self-trust because you're stating your authentic experience rather than pushing. If you're unsure which option feels right for you, just start reading Chapter Six. Allow the choice to unfold naturally – if you feel called to start practising and implementing, then go with option one. If you feel the chapter isn't resonating or is not right for you now, try option two.

One more option

There is one more option, by the way. One that may sound a little odd for me to suggest. If this all feels too much – if you can't take in any more information – simply read to the end of this chapter and stop. I want you to read the whole book, of course. But I want this less than I want you to be well. This chapter, along with the previous one, gives you an overview of trauma healing and building the four capacities. Although the detail is missing, the principles and theory are all covered. You now know what you need to do:

- Signal safety and learn to regulate.
- Become more present and curiously aware.
- Receive yourself with perspective and compassion.
- Acknowledge your agency and take self-led action.

So, if you feel overwhelmed, give yourself permission to stop reading, and instead, start putting these capacities into practice in a more instinctive and flexible way. Take the overarching *concepts* of each capacity and weave them into your day. Use the principles, too (page 156) to give a little more direction and structure to any self-led action you take. Come back to Chapters Six to Nine when you're ready for more guidance and learning.

Sneaky resistance

When our trauma and old patterning reacts to prevent change it's hard to spot (we believe and buy in to the whispered beliefs: you're getting this wrong, you need to start again, this isn't working, you're too unwell for this to work for you). Noticing the sneaky ways our trauma undermines our self-led choices is part of this journey. As you read the next four chapters, and implement the tools and principles, try to notice resistance, name it if you can, then signal safety and move back into self-led action (that is, keep reading!).

Action is the thing we always reach for. Inaction (the paralysis caused by all the self-doubt, self-mistrust and anxiety) is the thing we need to become increasingly aware of. Because adrenalised inaction is a sign we've been activated, and for that reason the story it's telling us reflects an old trauma-led script, not reality.

When to do deeper trauma work

This book opened with the line 'I'm not anti-therapy, but . . .' I'm really not anti-therapy. I love therapy. Arguably, I wouldn't be here without it. I just want the balance of power to shift so you can see and feel just how much power you have to create real change and deep healing by building capacity and resilience. Please, work with a therapist or practitioner, but know that you must also courageously take self-led action.

Although it's true that so much of this work is achieved through daily action to integrate capacities, it's also true that trauma healing often requires deeper work. By 'deeper work' I mean specific, intensive therapeutic work to help you process and release past traumas. Processing some emotion can be achieved through talking. But processing trauma memories and releasing intense trauma energy requires a mind-body approach, during which we slowly and safely contract (move into the trauma) and release (move into safety). This is because the imprint of the trauma exists in the body and the nervous system as well as the mind and psyche. The self-led approach offered in this book can achieve some gentle release and processing, but sometimes deeper work, facilitated by a practitioner, is needed.

To help me explain this concept, I spoke to Sheryl Close, a psychotherapist and consultant with decades of experience guiding people through deeper trauma work and into thriving. She specialises in trauma, addiction and eating disorders and is trained in advanced trauma resolution techniques such as Somatic Experiencing (SE), Somatic Regulation and Resilience (SRR) and Transforming Touch (TT). Before you dive into the self-led approach I want to share some of Sheryl's thoughts about possible signs that you'd benefit from working with a practitioner as you move through the four capacities:

Someone might need to do deeper work with a therapist if they continue to experience patterns that don't shift. These may be patterns in their thinking, emotions, behaviours, sensations, physical symptoms or relationships.

Also, if someone is having to consistently work hard and use techniques to try to calm themselves, it means they don't have enough regulation and capacity to make the self-led work they're doing stick and integrate. They may also have a continued inability to manage emotions when triggered, and either go into freeze or overwhelm.

Complex/developmental trauma may require a variety of modalities to allow a full healing. A somatic regulation-based modality such as Transforming Touch decreases an individual's nervous system dysregulation, bringing more emotional and psychological capacity. This allows other modalities including EMDR and IFS, as well as self-led work, to assimilate and therefore integrate and create lasting change.

Sheryl is rightly pointing out that if you are struggling to create change and take self-led action, it doesn't mean you lack willpower. It's simply a sign that co-regulation (regulating with another human) may be needed to *facilitate* self-regulation.

Remember Sheryl's words as you move into self-led healing. If you cannot create any movement or loosen a pattern or if you have to work very hard to regulate long term, consider working with a therapist or practitioner to support your self-led journey. Sheryl also highlighted some other, more extreme 'red-flag' signs that deeper trauma processing is needed. To find this information, please head to Chapter Ten, page 314.

The Principles of Self-led Integration

I've previously mentioned the Principles of Self-led Integration. Following and practising these principles as you take action is essential. They are the foundation of the capacities – whichever capacity you're building or technique you're practising, keep coming back to the principles. I've included reminders in the following chapters when a principle is especially relevant. Over time, these principles will become second nature – they're your new map, designed to help you move through life in a new, self-led, way. Here they are:

- Principle One: Stretch don't stress.
- Principle Two: Experiment and play to find what works.
- Principle Three: Repeat, repeat, repeat.
- Principle Four: Dip in and out of discomfort.
- Principle Five: Find your way back to green.
- Principle Six: Observe with curiosity.
- Principle Seven: Respond with compassion.
- Principle Eight: Anchored connection heals us.
- Principle Nine: Acknowledge your agency.
- Principle Ten: Allow your inner wisdom to guide you.
- Principle Eleven: Find soft places to land.

These principles have brought deep healing and real change to me and my clients. They're derived from the newer trauma modalities and theories – Internal Family Systems (IFS), Poly-vagal Theory, and Somatic Experiencing, and new research into neuroplasticity. Woven together, they create a powerful playbook for trauma healing.

Principle One: Stretch don't stress

This principle guides the self-led approach. Building sustainable trauma healing from the bottom up requires us to take a slow-and-steady approach to integrating the capacities we need. One per cent more of a capacity is still more.

Do not push yourself to do too much too soon or you'll move back into survival mode. This principle reminds us that our goal of creating a new way of being and reacting is achieved as we stretch ourselves but do not power or push our way back into survival. Stretch, don't stress, your nervous system.

Principle Two: Experiment and play to find what works

You need to experience and practise what you're learning here to fully integrate it. Real-time practice in our day-to-day lives can feel uncomfortable because it requires us to be present and to make mistakes.

Like any aspect of self-healing, allowing ourselves to practise what we're learning is a skill we need to gently build. Give yourself permission to experiment and approach the tools and capacities playfully. The more lightly you can hold this approach, and the more mistakes you make as you put it all into practice, the better. This principle reminds us that lighthearted playfulness helps facilitate regulation and create sustainable change.

Principle Three: Repeat, repeat, repeat

For decades you've been practising and repeating patterns that don't serve you. You will need similar dedication to create and embed new patterns that do serve you! Nervous systems are full of glorious potential for healing and change, but to harness this power we must repeat actions that we want to integrate (such as signalling safety, developing curiosity, practising compassion and setting boundaries).

This doesn't require military consistency, just an overall intention to move towards and repeat what we want more of.

Principle Four: Dip in and out of discomfort

Somatic Experiencing (SE) has demonstrated that trauma healing happens at the level of the nervous system through a process of contraction and release/expansion. We put this into practice by allowing ourselves to be with (notice, feel) discomfort for short periods of time, and then moving back into comfort and safety. As we gently shift between discomfort and comfort, trauma energy and healing energy, pain and goodness, our system contracts and releases in a safe way. This concept is fundamental to trauma healing – it's the active process that will help you release and expand. This principle reminds us that trauma healing isn't about sitting in pain and discomfort, but instead it's achieved as we consciously move between discomfort to comfort.

Principle Five: Find your way back to green

Notice when you move into the 'orange' zone (fight, flight) or 'red' zone (freeze, fawn, collapse). Then, take action to signal safety to your nervous system and move yourself back towards the green zone (self-connection and regulation). Any action that creates a little more calm, comfort or sense of connection to your environment and the present moment will signal safety to your nervous system. Long exhales, wrapping yourself in a blanket, placing your hand on your heart, smiling, singing and humming are examples that work well for many people.

It takes time to learn how to find your way back to green, largely because you may not have much conscious, embodied sense of what *green* feels like. Allow yourself to experiment (Principle Two) to find what works for you and take it slow – 1 per cent more time in the green zone tomorrow is still more (Principle One: Stretch don't stress). This principle reminds us that the green zone (the regulation that exists underneath survival) is home base.

Principle Six: Observe with curiosity

Instead of 'evidence-gathering', judging, criticising or catastroph-ising, try to approach yourself, your reactions, your emotions, your thoughts, your choices, your past and your patterns with curiosity.

You are your new project. Seek to understand through curiosity, and regulation and healing will flow. Judging, catastrophising and criticising only moves us further into dysregulation and slows down healing. This principle reminds us that curiosity is a powerful springboard into neuroplasticity and real change.

Principle Seven: Respond with adult compassion

Trauma healing goes hand-in-hand with your capacity to show yourself grounded, adult compassion. This means internally responding to yourself and your reactions with presence, an adult's viewpoint that keeps things in perspective, and kindness. Over time we practise seeing, hearing, validating and reassuring ourselves and the younger parts of our psyche. This could sound like internally saying: 'I know you're feeling anxious and tense – it's okay, everyone feels anxious sometimes.'

There's no expectation that you'll wake up tomorrow and be infinitely compassionate with yourself. But perhaps tomorrow you can show yourself 1 per cent more adult compassion.

Principle Eight: Anchored connection heals us

Trauma creates disconnection from the present moment, our body, our sense of self, the environment around us, other people and the world. Healing comes as we slowly, safely, gently reconnect over time. We do this naturally as our body feels safer. But we can facilitate connection by anchoring back into the present moment, our body and the environment around us, for example, by moving into our senses, noticing what we can see, touch, hear, smell or taste, or noticing the movement of our ribs as we gently breathe.

Although anchored connection heals us, too much connection too soon is triggering. Even a little more connection in a day is enough to facilitate trauma healing.

Principle Nine: Acknowledge your agency

Most triggered reactions are accelerated by a sense that we're suddenly out of control – that we no longer have choice or agency. To bring relief we need to acknowledge our agency, because although much of what's happening may very well be largely out of our control, we have agency and choice about how we respond.

A simple way to practise this is pausing when you feel activated or triggered because something suddenly feels out of control. First respond internally with compassion – say something like, 'It's okay, everyone feels out of control sometimes.' Then internally acknowledge and affirm your own agency, which could sound like, 'I'm an adult and I have agency – I can choose how I respond and what I do next.' This principle reminds us that becoming aware of the things we can control and the choices available to us moves us towards the green zone and away from trauma.

Principle Ten: Allow your inner wisdom to guide you

As you move through the self-led approach you'll reconnect to your anchored adult self. This process is life-changing because it brings us back to our inner guidance system and wisdom.

It takes time to hear and feel the compassionate, wise voice of our adult self. As we move into regulation and curiosity, and as we become less enmeshed with our younger parts, we become able to slow down and connect, so we can hear our own inner source of wisdom.

Listen out for this moderate, compassionate, wise voice of adult reason. This is self, and it embodies the wisdom you will use to create rather than react.

Principle Eleven: Find soft places to land

Co-regulation, support and safe connection facilitate trauma healing. Everybody, no matter where we are in our healing journey, needs to be seen and understood by another. At times we all need reassurance – we need someone else's adult self to hold us when we're in our wounding.

Support facilitates healing *and* thriving. It builds resilience and flexibility in our nervous system. As you move through this self-led approach, find soft places to land. Whether this is, say, a psychologist, therapist, other practitioner, support group, friend or spiritual teacher, slowly start to build a team of people you feel safe (or safe enough) around. This principle reminds us that self-led does not mean alone.

Integrating the principles

These principles are the foundation of the four capacities and of trauma healing through sustainable change. You'll learn more about these principle as you read and implement the next four chapters. Here I've deliberately omitted detail so as not to give you formulaic instructions, but to inspire you. They're succinct ideas and concepts, as all principles need to be.

Take these ideas and allow them to percolate and expand within you. Make them your own. But also be reassured that if a principle feels a little too abstract, by the end of the book you'll have a deeper understanding of it.

Chapter Six

Capacity one: signalling safety and self-regulating

Embodying safety – learning how to help your beautiful body feel safer – is one of the four core capacities of trauma healing. Embodied safety *facilitates* deep healing and real change. If you've spent your whole life feeling disconnected from your body and unsafe, what I've just said may feel completely unattainable. Know you're not alone – most of us start this work with very little embodied experience of 'safe'. We, like you, don't know what the mountain top looks or feels like. Lacking an embodied experience of 'safe and comfortable' is normal in this world of trauma healing.

Just as you learned to ride a bike or read, you can learn how to feel safer in your body if you take it one day at a time. It's a capacity you can practise and develop. Much like everything you'll learn here, there's a knack to it. We slowly learn how to *signal safety* to our nervous system via our ventral vagal nerve, and as we do we move into regulation. Over time we create a new neural map, and as we rewire our nervous system, our experience of life changes.

Childhood trauma leaves our nervous system on high alert for noticing threats. Childhood trauma *healing*, then, is about signalling to our nervous system that we are now safe. We move from subconsciously noticing threats in our environment, mind and body to consciously noticing safety in our environment and inner world. Learning to signal safety even during moments of stress overrides and interrupts our old conditioning. It's simple, basic neuroscience, and it works. Your 'there's a threat' response has become habitual through years of overuse. As you interrupt these pathways and create new conditioned responses, you'll begin to have a very different experience of life.

There are many ways to signal safety to your nervous system and a lot of them are very obvious. The things you would intuitively presume might help you feel a bit safer are likely to be the things your nervous system picks up on as an objective sign of safety. Being in nature, smiling, mindful slow movement, deepening your breathing, giving yourself a cuddle and connecting with safe people or animals are all pretty obvious (and effective) ways to signal to your nervous system that you're safe.

Having said this, as Julia Samuel highlighted in the previous chapter, following 'shoulds' as you build this capacity will not serve you. Do you remember I told you that Fiona tasked me with doing nothing? This *should* have felt good, right? There I was, 'signalling safety to my nervous system' by anchoring into my senses and the present moment and it didn't feel good at all. It was torturous. My nervous system believed that the present moment was deeply threatening for me. I couldn't just be present. This was very useful information for me at that point. It helped me see that I had to build my capacity to be present, and it took a very long time. At that time, doing nothing didn't help me feel safer. It didn't feel good. I had to find other ways. Please remember this bizarre image of me attempting to 'do nothing' as you explore what feels good. Don't follow a 'should' – follow what feels genuinely comfortable to your body. And follow these simple rules:

- If it feels too much, stop.
- If it feels better/comfortable/tolerable/lovely, keep going *and* do it more often.

Before we move on, take some time to experience the concept of signalling safety by trying these three short practices. Take your time with these exercises. Slow them down. See if you can experience them from within your body – try to anchor your mind into your body, its sensations and its movements. Even if you're in your body and aware of the sensations for just a few seconds, that's a win. Try to notice which (if any) feel good and bring a sense of relief or ease. Also try to be aware if any of the exercises create more discomfort and *less* safety.

Practice One (touch): You can signal a little more safety to your body right now by putting your hand on your heart and rubbing and patting your chest as you would to soothe a child. You could close your eyes and say to yourself, 'It's okay, you're safe.' Keep doing this until you feel a little sense of release. You might even notice that you exhale more deeply, releasing tension from your body.

Practice Two (imagination): For this one you need to be sitting in a chair. Close your eyes if that feels safe and comfortable. Exhale deep and long, and as you do, drop your shoulders and imagine yourself leaning back onto a big rock that has been warmed by the sun. Feel its sturdiness behind you. Allow it to hold you and warm you. Breathe slowly and deeply, while picturing the support behind you, and observe what happens in your body and emotions as you do.

Practice Three (movement): Next, try rocking from side to side, either seated or standing, finding a rhythm and a flow – just as a mother rocks a newborn baby. Experiment with whether having your eyes open or closed feels more comfortable. Notice any shifts in how you are feeling. Do this for as long as you need, particularly if it feels good and soothing.

These three exercises are ones I've used often over the years. They're simple and work well for many people. If one of them worked well for you – if it worked to 'signal safety' to your nervous system – add it to your toolbox. The more you use it the more effectively it'll work to help you feel safer and bring you back into connection with your body, environment and self.

Self-led integration: A reminder

You're about to read a great number of tools and techniques, all of which can be used to move you into regulation and embodied safety. Although the tools *can* be used to self-regulate, en masse they can also be overwhelming. Please hear me when I say: you do not need to learn every technique. To build this capacity, aim to use one or two tools a day. The tools you initially choose may be ones you're still using months later – they may become part of your toolbox. Or, you may find yourself experimenting as time goes on. There's no right way to do this and the only 'wrong' way to do it is not to do anything at all.

Choose tools or techniques that you're naturally drawn to or that feel easy. Most people find the imagination techniques (page 182) and the soothing and activation techniques (page 185) easier to get started with than the anchoring techniques (page 189).

As you begin to practise this capacity, remember *how* we integrate – daily action and repetition. To build this capacity, take daily action to signal safety to your nervous system. This move from activation to balance is self-regulation. Repeat your chosen action, or actions, multiple times a day. The individual techniques you choose matter less than the act of repeating 'signalling safety and regulating'. You can do this using different tools and techniques each time.

As well as daily action and repetition, we integrate by reminding ourselves of the foundations of self-led healing – the Principles of Self-led Integration. In particular, as you practise this first capacity, remember principles One, Two and Three:

- Principle One: Stretch don't stress.
- Principle Two: Experiment and play to find what works.
- Principle Three: Repeat, repeat, repeat.

Stretch yourself a little each day, but don't stress yourself by setting unrealistic goals – remember, 1 per cent more is enough

(Principle One). Give yourself permission to play around with different techniques to find which works best for you (Principle Two). Signal safety multiple times a day and over the long term. Remember, it takes 254 days to rewire complex actions, so aim for compassionate consistency to ensure these behaviours become a new way of living (Principle Three).

The Capacity One Polarities

Although I'm always trying to help clients move out of black-and-white thinking, I've noticed that using polarities to explain the journey from trauma to healing is extremely helpful for many. A polarity comprises two things that are polar opposites. Hot and cold are polarities, as are war and peace. The clarity and simplicity of these divisions helps us understand what we're moving from and to. The polarities that will help you better understand Capacity One are:

- Dysregulated vs regulated
- Disembodied vs embodied
- Signalling threat vs signalling safety
- Expansion vs protection
- Autopilot vs action
- Detached vs anchored
- Contraction vs release
- Disconnected vs connected

A conversation

There are a multitude of ways to signal safety to your nervous system and help you move into the ventral vagal zone of regulation (the green zone). There's no bad time to do this – the more time you spend in the green zone, the better. It's also true that over time we want to move into a *conversation* with our nervous system and body. This means developing the skill of noticing when we're moving into dysregulation and then taking action to help ourselves move towards regulation and balance. We become responsive and flexible, and able to create movement in our nervous system, rather than being stuck in survival and autopilot.

Learning to self-regulate, then, isn't about never getting stressed, anxious, triggered or overwhelmed. It's about being able to bring ourselves and our system back into balance after stress. Self-regulation is rhythm. We notice we've moved into dysregulation – into stress, contraction, striving, endurance, anxiety, fear and so on – and then take action to move ourselves back in to (or towards) the green zone. Down and up, up and down. As we do this, we move out of trauma-led patterns and into self-led patterns. Remember also that, when applied mindfully, each of the eleven principles will move you towards the green zone.

Notice

The first part of learning to self-regulate is noticing when you're moving into survival. To do this, you need to get really really curious about your own signs of dysregulation because the earlier you spot it, the less likely it is that you'll move into a full-on triggered reaction. Think about it now. How do you know you're moving into fight, flight, freeze, fawn or collapse? Are you fast and racy? Breathing in a shallow way? Anxious? Obsessing? Overwhelmed? Confused? Afraid? Irritable? Angry? Overreacting? Avoiding people? Picking your nails? Dissociating and starting to float away? Overthinking? Has your mind moved into catastrophic thinking? Are you panicking you've said something wrong? Unable to focus? Feeling 'less than'? Has your stomach dropped and that foggy feeling of shame come over you? Can you relate or are these just mine?!

The first step is noticing that you're moving into the orange (fight, flight) or red (freeze, fawn, collapse) zone, then getting curious about how these states affect your thinking, your body, your emotions and your behaviours. Over time, you want to build up a picture of how you experience these different nervous system states. This takes time and depends on you becoming increasingly able to notice what's going on in your body, mind and behaviour. We're aiming to slowly move from a disembodied, disconnected, unconscious, protective way of living into an embodied, connected, conscious way of living. Practising Capacity Two (moving into awareness) will support this, but it's something we naturally also start practising as we integrate Capacity One.

We do this by noticing our discomfort – we become aware of and allow ourselves to be with the discomfort for a moment. For example, noticing the sudden contraction of our chest and our shallow breathing in response to something that feels threatening or too much. To help lessen the intensity we can then label it anxiety or fear. We could also add some grounded adult compassion by saying to yourself, 'It's okay, everyone feels anxious sometimes.' The 'noticing' step, then, is about connecting with what is real for us as we move into discomfort, with an energy of curiosity and compassion.

See Diagram 4 for common signs of dysregulation and survival, mapped onto what can be thought of as the green, orange and red zones. Take your time with this chart – notice how the nervous system's survival states impact so much more than our body. Signs you need to take action to move towards the green zone (the bottom third of the chart) are diverse and affect our mind and behaviour as much as our body and emotions (for example, they can be expressed as confusion or procrastination).

We also need to develop an embodied sense of how it feels to be in the green zone as we build up this picture of how the orange (middle third) and red (top third) zones feel. As I've said before, most of us come to this work without a clear sense of what regulation and self feel like. As we practise self-led healing, we begin to get a sense of contrast between comfortable and uncomfortable, activated and not activated. Get as curious about how the green zone feels as you are about what happens when you move into the orange and red zones.

Respond

The second part of learning to self-regulate is doing what you can to create more ease and comfort in your body. Signalling safety so you feel even 1 per cent less activated is a win. Literally, that's it: this conversation happens as you notice and then take self-led action.

Self-regulation isn't complicated, but it takes a long time to fully integrate this capacity. To begin with, everything can feel messy and extreme, and it's hard to differentiate states and responses. Finding the response that brings relief also takes time and practice. As we increasingly connect to our bodies, we notice we're becoming activated earlier, so we respond earlier. There's also more space between us and our reactions. Everything feels slower and easier to handle. But not to start with. To start with, self-regulation can feel odd, uncomfortable and challenging. So be gentle with yourself as you begin this important self-led work.

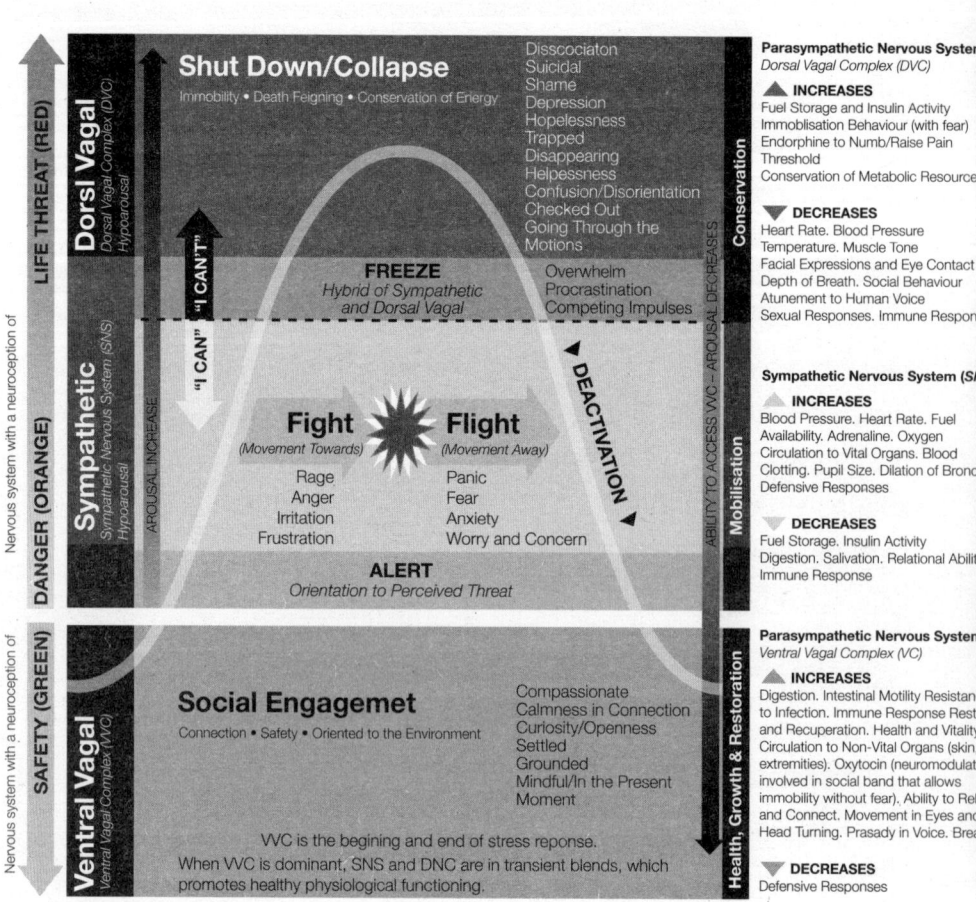

Diagram 4: Polyvagal Theory Chart of Trauma Response
© Ruby Jo Walker, LCSW 2018 • Southwest Trauma Training • swtraumatraining.com • Adapted by Ruby Jo Walker from Cheryl Sanders, Dr Peter Levine, Anthony 'Twig' Wheeler, and Dr Stephen Porges

Self-regulation: yin and yang

Self-regulation illustrates the concept of yin and yang: where two opposite forces are interconnected and complementary. Trauma creates imbalance in the nervous system – we develop rigid patterns of dysregulation. Healing means learning how to create more balance – allowing us to flexibly move back into regulation. This requires us to either switch on parasympathetic rest and repair energy by signalling safety to our nervous system, and/or release sympathetic arousal energy by allowing the biological impulse to complete and discharge. Most often we need to do both. Focusing on only one is likely to compound our sense of imbalance over time.

As you integrate Capacity One, remember the concept of yin and yang. Embodying safety isn't just about calming or down-regulating our nervous systems (as described in the previous section), it also requires us to 'up-regulate' by moving and releasing arousal energy – at times we must shout, cry, shake, stamp. Both the yin and yang of self-regulation increase our sense of embodied safety because both bring more ease and comfort to our body.

Meet yourself where you're at

The four capacities of trauma healing are all interlinked – so much so that it was hard to decide which to explain first. I've landed here: the capacity to signal safety, because it is so foundational. But before we dive in, I need to make it very clear that because this isn't a linear process, different things will work for different people at different times. To illustrate this point, I want to share with you something a client, Naomi, said to me recently:

> When you first told me about all the somatic [body] stuff I genuinely didn't get it. I know you said it would help but in all honesty I didn't really understand how to actually *do* anything you suggested. I was doubtful, suspicious and reluctant. I spent my entire life trying to *think* my way out of having to actually *feel* and whenever I got too close to genuine feeling, my habitual resistance

kicked in. Now I know I simply wasn't ready to connect to and actively focus on my body (the thing I'd been avoiding for forty years).

I first focused on pretty much anything other than looking closely at what was going on in my body. I focused on understanding my trauma patterns, becoming more present in daily life and learning how to reassure and support myself in a new way. I think this all helped me feel safer in my body without me having to directly *do* somatic work!

Six months ago, and three years into this journey, I started actively focusing on connecting to and healing my body. I just knew it was time. I used Deb Dana and Peter Levine's somatic exercises. They helped me become aware of my body's sensations in a totally new way.

Finally learning how to work with my somatic sensations and connect to the wisdom of my physical body completely changed my experience of life and my understanding of my trauma. But I had to do it when I was ready.

Today Naomi is thriving, present and in flow. She has a profound connection to her body and to her sense of adult self. She is curious, compassionate and self-led. She is remarkable, as so many of my clients are. Three years after first approaching me to help her heal her childhood trauma, Naomi was ready to actively look at, be in and soothe her body. She could not have done this a moment earlier. Her story illustrates the importance of giving yourself permission to instinctively guide your journey.

So, give yourself permission now to *feel* your way through this chapter. If some of this *body stuff* feels too much, move on.

There's no 'right' way to integrate the four capacities, so if you need to, follow Naomi's example and confidently move onto Capacity Two, then come back to the more body-focused work when you feel ready.

The power of your imagination to signal safety

Naomi's story demonstrates the power of going slowly and meeting ourselves where we're at – doing what feels right, and what we *can* do, rather than what we 'should' do. As Naomi practised and developed capacities Two and Three she signalled safety to her body and moved into regulation. Focusing on these capacities first was a gentle way in to self-regulation for Naomi. But there's one part of her story I haven't mentioned that I think you need to hear. Before Naomi learned how to signal safety in real life, soothing and reassuring herself in real time when things were challenging, she first experienced this in her *imagination*. Yes, you heard me right.

Every morning for six months Naomi spent time in what she called her 'mother garden'. This was a safe space she created mentally, a space in which she felt completely relaxed and protected.

Over time, and with practice, she found she could access this space, with its associated feeling of safety and regulation, more and more easily. Even after stressful or challenging events, she would imagine herself in this place surrounded by nature, nourishment and comfort. As time went on, Naomi also imagined a mother figure sitting in this garden alongside her. Being in this imagined place of peace, and with this wise, unconditionally loving adult, signalled a very real sense of safety to Naomi's nervous system and body.

Naomi's story illustrates a profound but simple truth: our imagination is one of the most powerful self-led tools we have at our disposal to signal safety to our nervous system. This may sound odd, but this truth is based firmly in fact because the nervous system cannot tell the difference between what's happening right now and what's happening in our imagination. As far as her nervous system is concerned, Naomi really did spend an hour a day in this safe, nourishing mother garden.

Another client, Charlotte, used her imagination in a very different but equally powerful way. In the past, Charlotte experienced multiple traumatic medical procedures, so part of her was now terrified by the thought of accompanying her daughter to an upcoming medical procedure. In the run-up to the appointment, Charlotte visualised the outcome she wanted. Every day for two weeks she pictured herself feeling calm and regulated as she got into the car to drive to the hospital. She pictured herself and her daughter laughing and joking. She pictured entering the hospital feeling light and joyful, with the sun shining on them both. She pictured cuddling her daughter as she came around from surgery, laughing and smiling together and feeling grateful that it went well. This visualisation lasted just 90 seconds – but Charlotte *felt* every single moment of it as if it was real. By the time she had to take her daughter to the hospital, Charlotte had visualised the experience over 40 times. On the day she felt little anxiety, no panic and a new sense of safety. The experience of being in a hospital was radically different for Charlotte – she had used her imagination to interrupt old patterns and create the felt experience she longed for.

To illustrate this further, let me tell you a little about my own experience. It's bizarrely true that initially, in the aftermath of the MS diagnosis, the only safe way for me to action changes was in my imagination. Although I ran most days in the rain-forest next to my home, probably more interesting is that I also ran every day, in my mind. I visualised myself leaping from rock to rock, seeing myself coming to a clearing high up in the forest, standing arms outstretched and bathed in light. I saw myself arriving back in England, walking confidently through Heathrow airport smiling and laughing.

I pictured light flowing through my nervous system, mind and body like a wave – breathing light in through my feet, watching it flow up and down my body, healing and nourishing as it did so. Every day I pictured specific areas of my nervous system healing – woven back together by a golden thread of light. Every day, literally every single day, I pictured the future I wanted: a neurologist showing me a scan that revealed that the MS had healed. I felt these moments as if they were real – experiencing the joy as if I was in that doctor's office being delivered the good of an already-healthy nervous system.

Why did I inhabit this odd fantasy world on a daily basis? The simple answer is: because it felt good and not much else did. But I was also aware of the mounting evidence within neuroscience research that our nervous system can't tell the difference between what is real and what is imagined. I understood, intellectually at least, that I could use my imagination to increase my sense of safety and regulation and therefore help my body move into healing. During these imaginary moments my body relaxed, my heart rate slowed and I felt hope rising. I also had a sense that I was connecting to something greater than myself – a healing power that existed within me and around me.

It's often said that 'hope heals us.' I believe this with all my heart. After the diagnosis, I intuitively understood that I had to find something to put my faith in, something to trust and lean on. If I didn't find a glimmer of hope and a whisper of something beautiful, the fear would engulf me, the stress would continue to rise and my body would become sicker. I chose to trust the healing power of the mind, body and spirit. And, no matter how anxious, unwell or defeated you feel, no matter how low trauma, illness, addiction or crisis has pulled you, I hope you can come to trust this too.

Perhaps asking you to trust the healing power of your mind, body and spirit feels too much of a leap? If it does, perhaps you can become willing to trust the *possibility* that you can heal. Just a little bit of openness, a little bit of curiosity, is all that's necessary to move into growth and away from survival.

I no longer spend hours visualising healing. But I have to mention this work that I diligently, silently, purposefully undertook daily for nearly eighteen months because it got me through an intensely tough time. My mind and body have experienced the conversation with the doctor about 547 times. It's now part of my inner world, because I put it there. These gentle, beautiful visualisations created a deep sense of empowerment and self-efficacy within me. They helped me move from fear of the unknown to faith in myself and my body. They created a profound sense of hope and self-trust, and for this reason helped me move out of a chronic state of dysregulation into regulation.

Imagination and the nervous system

The visualisation practices I relied on in the aftermath of the MS diagnosis may sound bizarre, but like my whole approach, they work because they're evidence-based. Your nervous system is magical, but it's not otherworldly or mystical. It's right there, waiting for you to learn how to harness its healing power. Once you understand the language of the nervous system, once you can speak to it and shape it, you can and will heal.

The lead fact here is that your nervous system cannot tell the difference between what's happening in reality and what's happening in your imagination. It will respond to, say, you *imagining* that you are safely snuggled up in a duvet as if you really are. There are some rules to this type of mind-body imagining, though. We must feel it, see it and be in it as much as we can. We slow things down and notice our imaginary world. We don't just whizz through it while doing the washing-up. It must be an emotional (whole-body) experience, not just a thought process.

You can experience a simple example of this if you now close your eyes and imagine (*really* imagine – see it, feel it, taste it) sucking a lemon. Even though there's no lemon on your tongue, your nervous system responds to your mind and you'll feel your tastebuds react and your mouth tighten. Weird.

The opposite is also true, by the way. Picture danger and your nervous system will respond as if you are indeed in danger. For this reason I confidently tell clients that, yes, nightmares can be traumatic. If you've run from a lion all night you have, in many ways, run from a lion all night.

In 2004, a team of scientists in Ohio explored the benefits of an *imaginary* strength training program. For 12 weeks, one group of men did strength exercises for real and another group *imagined* they were doing the same strength exercises. Muscle gain in the group who were doing 15 minutes a day of imaginary training went up 35 per cent (finger strength) and 13.5 per cent (bicep strength).[1] These results blow my mind! Simply imagining that we're doing exercise activates the nervous system and leads to muscle gain.

In *You Are the Placebo*, Dr Joe Dispenza describes multiple studies that illustrate that the imagination, thought and belief may have a huge impact on biology. He describes a 2001 study conducted by scientist Raúl Fuente-Fernández and his colleagues, in which the researchers told a group of Parkinson's patients that they would receive a drug that would significantly improve their symptoms. In reality, patients received a placebo – a saline injection. Despite this, over 50 per cent of the group had better motor control after receiving the injection. The researchers scanned the patients' brains to understand what was going on and saw that those with improved motor control had up to 200 per cent more dopamine than before the injection. In other words, simply expecting to get better led to a huge increase in dopamine (which the body needs to heal), which in turn may have led to improved motor control.[2]

To understand more about how different clinicians use the imagination to facilitate trauma healing, I interviewed Lou Lebentz, a psychotherapist and EMDR practitioner with decades of clinical experience. She is funny, engaging and kind. As a real-life example of just how kind Lou is: she sat with me for nearly two hours answering a multitude of questions about her approach to trauma healing. Here's what Lou shared about how EMDR practitioners use a client's imagination to create more safety and regulation:

At the very start of treatment I install *a safe enough place* in a client's imagination – an imagined place where they can feel safe enough. *Enough* is the operative word because most trauma survivors never feel *fully* safe anywhere. If it's a real place, it has to be free of any memory where there was any sort of dysregulation or unsafe *other*.

Then we install nurturing figures, wise figures and protector figures. They could be animals, they could be superheroes, they could be Nelson Mandela or Gandalf. It doesn't matter. You could put somebody's best friend, you could put symbols, you could put an energetic field that feels like it's a safe object. Anything that helps regulate them. Then, in day-to-day life, they can imagine that those figures are with them.

The language Lou uses is specific to the EMDR framework. In lay terms, Lou is simply using a client's imagination to create and install images in the mind that simultaneously feel good and safe. It's about using the imagination to positively affect a client's body and move them towards embodied safety and regulation.

All trauma practitioners, no matter which discipline they've trained in, use the imagination to increase regulation and signal safety to the nervous system. The imagination is used in other ways too. When practitioners do deeper trauma work that involves traumatic beliefs or memories from the past, they use the imagination to reframe, process and change the 'emotional imprint' of the memory. The imagination is used to facilitate the active trauma healing process of contraction and release. When done in a safe, whole-body way, *imagining* standing up for ourselves or fighting back, say, can create a profound sense of resolution. As neuroscientist Marianne Cumella Reddan says:

If you have a memory that is no longer useful for you or is crippling you, you can use imagination to tap into it, change it and re-consolidate it, updating the way you think about and experience something.[3]

Your imagination is one of the most powerful self-led tools you have at your disposal. Doing this work with a practitioner is powerful, but remember that it's *your* imagination. You can use it any minute of the day to signal safety to your nervous system and move your body into rest and repair.

Imagination techniques

My hope is that you now have a greater sense of appreciation for the power of your imagination to signal safety to your nervous system. In Appendix B I describe two visualisations that work well for most of my clients. The first is a safe space visualisation, similar to those installed in an initital EMDR session. The second is a healing light visualisation – similar to the one I used for those eighteen months. Head to page 320 to find these. You can also download audios of both mind-body visualisations for free at my website (sarahwoodhouse.com). Remember though, these visualisations are just suggestions. The power of your imagination is truly unlimited.

The ventral vagal nerve

Signalling safety to our nervous system is all about learning the language of the *ventral vagal pathway* of the vagus nerve (for an overview of this nerve see page 14). When the ventral vagal pathway senses safety and activates we feel:

- Flexible and responsive
- Open and curious

- Anchored and connected
- Present
- Compassionate.

A well-functioning ventral vagal nerve means we can tolerate small daily stresses and hiccups without moving into survival mode. We're able to self-regulate – moving from arousal to rest in a flexible way. It also means that we're moving into rest and repair, meaning that our body can begin to heal. In the previous few sections I explained how the imagination can be used to activate the ventral vagal pathway. Now I want to talk about more concrete action you can take to signal safety to your nervous system. Lou Lebentz describes this beautifully:

Regulation happens as we come back into the ventral vagal green zone, so I'm always getting clients to practise what brings them back up to green. Their safe enough place is going to bring them back, but so are their positive beliefs about themselves, their dog or their walk in nature. Whether it's swimming, whether it's horse riding, whether it's phoning a friend, whether it's a particular food they eat or putting a blanket over themselves and watching a favourite episode of *Friends* on Netflix. There are regulatory things that they can put into practice on a daily basis to get their nervous system a bit more *into the green*!

Remember Lou's words as you start to explore ways to signal safety to your nervous system – moving into the green zone is simply about becoming aware of things that feel genuinely good and safe for us.

There are two top-level ways to signal safety to the body via the ventral vagal nerve. The first involves activating the nerve using specific techniques that soothe and signal safety. The second is through deepening your sense of anchored connection with the present moment, your body, your adult self, your environment and other people. Many of the techniques I describe here, including the imagination techniques above, both soothe and anchor in one way or another. But I find this distinction helpful for many clients. As you practise signalling safety, use a mix of tools to soothe and activate the ventral nerve, alongside tools to anchor and connect you to your body and the world around you.

Ventral vagal as self

Before we move into the techniques, I want to remind you of the importance, the magic, of what we're doing here. As you interrupt trauma-led patterns of threat and intentionally self-regulate to widen your window of tolerance and signal safety, you are connecting back to *self*.

Understanding the concept of our self in terms of the nervous system is pretty simple. Our adult self *emerges* as we move towards regulation and ventral activation. Think about the five facets of ventral vagal activation I've just listed: flexibility and responsiveness, openness and curiosity, anchoring and connection, presence and compassion. It's from this state of regulation that we can know ourselves – our values, needs and wants. As we move into this state we move out of trauma and old conditioning. We become free. This state, then, is where our true agency and power lie – because it's here that we can know ourselves and see reality.

Your journey through trauma healing and self-led integration is a journey back to self. As you build each capacity, you'll experience self in different ways – as awareness, as a wise, loving adult, as empowered action. Here, in Capacity One, self is experienced as a flexible nervous system state or energy that we learn to move into. This concept isn't the whole picture, but it's the foundation of an authentic, aligned sense of self that can direct your life and create real change.

Soothing and activation techniques

1. **Resonant breathing:** make your exhalations the same length as your inhalations.
   Inhale for a slow count of four, pause, then exhale for a slow count of four.
2. **Polyvagal breathing:** extend your exhalations.
   Place one hand on your heart and one on your diaphragm, taking slow breaths down into your belly. Resting your hand on your diaphragm will help you notice the movement of your breath. Inhale into your belly like this for four counts, pause at the fourth count and exhale for six counts. After a few of these breath cycles, extend the exhalation further – inhale for four, hold for four, exhale for eight.
3. **Physiological sigh:** the double inhale or 'double-bump' breath.
   At the top of your inhale, take another, shorter inhale. Effectively, you inhale twice: the first to about 80 per cent lung capacity, the second the last 20 per cent. Hold for a count of two then exhale very, very slowly while dropping your shoulders and relaxing your body. Do this at least three times.

4. **Embody ventral energy:** adopt a ventral posture.
    This is a lovely one and it works well for many clients. Stand tall, with a straight posture, shoulders back and loose, feet hip-width apart and smile. Doing this helps your body learn how it feels to be in the green zone, even if you aren't there yet emotionally.

5. **Slow down:** as simple as it sounds!
    Really exaggerate this – whatever you are doing, move as slowly as you can. A popular form of this exercise is the Buddhist meditation technique of 'mindful walking', where you walk as slowly as possible around the room, really taking in every detail of every step, noticing how you place your feet and the subtle movements of your body as you shift weight from right to left.

6. **Rosenberg technique:** occipital bone release.
    This takes practice and can be easier to do with a partner; it basically involves releasing tension from the neck muscles at the bottom of your skull using finger pressure. See Appendix F for full instructions and reference. This technique works well for many of my clients. It releases tension, signals safety, activates the ventral nerve and moves us into our social engagement system.

7. **Bilateral stimulation:** eye movement.
    With your head facing forward, look to the left for twenty seconds. Next, relax and look straight ahead for couple of seconds. Now move your gaze to the right for twenty seconds. It can help to use your fingers to fix your gaze – hold your finger to the left and follow it with your eyes, then move it to the centre, then to the right, following with your eyes each time. Do this four times. This exercise is believed to help you integrate the right and left

hemispheres of your brain, which is integral to regulation and trauma healing as it brings emotion and cognition into balance.

8. **Vibration:** voooo.

Inhale deeply into the belly and exhale as slowly as you can, using a 'voooooooooooooooo' sound. Once you have exhaled all the way out, allow the next breath to come in naturally, then repeat the sound again. Keep repeating as many times as you need, noticing the sensations in your body as you do it. This exercise stimulates the vagus nerve, helping you to feel more settled.

9. **Vibration:** hum or sing.

Humming or singing vibrates the throat, which stimulates the vagal nerve. Hum or sing anything you want! Don't worry if you think you 'can't sing' – this is not about making music, but about regulating your nervous system.

10. **Rhythmical movement:** swaying, circling hips, bobbing, slow dancing.

Rhythm feels safe to the body and nervous system, so any rhythmical movement can move you out of dorsal vagal activation – the red zone of freeze/collapse – and towards the green zone – ventral vagal activation, where you feel regulated and safe.

11. **Self-touch:** cuddle, stroke, massage.

Safe touch can be very soothing. Don't overthink this – touch your body in a way that feels nice – give yourself a cuddle, cover your eyes with your hands, rub your neck, give your feet a rub, squeeze your calf muscles. Our bodies evolved to calm down when we are touched with care, and it's something we can provide for ourselves even if we didn't receive it in childhood.

The knack to these techniques is that you need to do them until you feel a little shift – sensing your energy/body changing in a positive way. You may notice that you sigh, yawn or take a deeper inhale; that your stomach gurgles, or that you simply feel *a little better* as the parasympathetic ventral branch switches on. It's also totally okay if you don't notice a shift – trust that as you practise these tools over time and deepen your connection to your body, you will.

Anchoring and connection

Trauma disconnects us from many things. When we're triggered, we're thrown back into an old reaction and a younger, wounded part of us takes over. We quite literally disconnect from the present moment as our survival response moves us into fight-flight, freeze, fawn or collapse. Trauma healing is all about reconnection. This idea – that connection heals us – is essential to what we're doing here. It's one of the Principles of Self-led Integration. It's your north star: connection is the mountain top. All four of the trauma healing capacities, and every single tool I present in this book, are designed to increase your connection to either the present moment, your body, your adult self, your environment and/or other people.

As we gently reconnect in a slow, self-led way, we feel safer. The reconnection anchors us and interrupts old trauma-led patterns. Signalling safety, then, is all about anchoring into the present moment and to little pockets of safety that exist in reality. We're looking for moments of connection that bring us into the green zone. This is a weird old journey, though, because too much connection too soon feels overwhelming and triggering. So we must take it slowly, always remembering to stretch but not stress our nervous system. It is essential to apply Principle Four – dipping in and out of discomfort. Movement is everything here – we don't want to remain in anything intense for long.

Below are different types of connection for you to start weaving into your day. First I describe anchoring techniques – ways you can anchor into the present moment via your mind and body. Next I describe nourishing ways of signalling safety through connection to the world around you. Practise the anchoring techniques first, as you'll use these, along with the soothing and activation techniques, to help you feel safe during real-world moments of connection. For example, anchor into your body when you're around other people to help signal safety to yourself.

Anchoring techniques

Anchoring through your senses

This is about receiving sensory information in a really gentle way. Don't search for information (this way of perceiving maintains fight/flight). Look at your environment with a soft gaze and allow the colours to come to you. Listen to the birds, simply allowing the sound to arrive at your ears without striving to hear it. Smell the grass, or your cup of coffee, taking gentle inhales. Gently touch a blanket and notice the softness. Receive the information, don't strain. A more structured way to do this is the 'three, two, one' exercise, in which you slowly name three things you can see, two you can hear and one you can touch. It can be helpful to repeat the phrase 'I am home' or 'I am safe' as you re-anchor into your environment and the present moment.

Anchoring into goodness

This type of connection helps us slowly alter our perception and combat our hypervigilance. Seek out, name, notice and expand things that feel good and safe. For example, perhaps your tummy feels full, comfortable and warm. If so, let your body know that you're receiving its safety signals – pause and really pay attention. Or perhaps your blanket feels soft and comforting. Again, be with those sensations and note them to yourself, almost as if you're making a mental note of just how good and safe the blanket feels. If you're enjoying this connection, see if you can expand the good, safe feelings – lean into them, really feel them, allow yourself to smile if you feel like it. This type of connection is similar to connecting to the environment through your senses, but the emphasis is on seeking out and feeling good/safe things around us or within us – the wind in the trees, the sun on our skin, the colours of our favourite mug and so on.

Anchoring into your body

Reconnection to our body requires us to increasingly be in and with our body. Over time, our body once again becomes our anchor. Self-touch is a soothing way to re-establish connection to the body, as I described on page 187. Mindful breathing, focusing on the movement of your ribs or belly, or the flow of air in and out of your nostrils, as you use resonant breathing, and body scans (moving your attention slowly through your body) are also gentle ways to reconnect. Yoga nidra and non-sleep deep rest (NSDR) recordings guide you through a combination of mindfulness and body scans. I explain these practices in more detail on page 209. Many clients use these audios multiple times a day to reconnect to their body, activate their ventral vagal nerve and move into regulation. See Appendix C for some links to good resources where you can find these recordings.

Dropping your attention down into your body as you go through the day is a powerful way of connecting and anchoring. We simply pause, drop our attention down to, say, our heart space, belly, sit bones or feet and then be here, breathing and connecting for a few seconds. This type of moment-by-moment connection (moving back into the body, and therefore, the present moment) is an essential part of the new way of life you're moving into. Begin practising this anchoring during more neutral moments, for example while drinking a cup of tea. Play with this. When you feel comfortable with this movement, explore how it feels to move down into your body during moments of stress. Many find this anchoring particularly comforting during social situations that can feel too much.

Being in our body involves connecting to emotions or sensations that may feel uncomfortable, so we take it slowly and apply the Principles of Self-led Integration (in particular Four, Five, Six and Seven).

Real-world connection techniques

Although it's theoretically true that being in nature, around animals, and around other people *should* signal safety, for those with childhood trauma the opposite is often the case. Remember to use the anchoring techniques and the soothing and/or activation techniques as you begin to explore forming nourishing real-world connections. We signal safety (using the anchoring and activation techniques) during real-world experiences so we can have a different, more nourishing type of connection. This takes time and practice, so go slow and remember Principle Three – we unlock the power of neuro-plasticity through repetition combined with compassion and curiosity.

Connect to nature

Even if you can't be outside, you can feel the sun on your skin through the window, watch the trees and the birds, or open the window and feel the breeze on your skin. If you can, go outside. Walk in nature or sit in nature. Take your shoes off if you can. Feel the earth under your feet. Slow things down so you can soak in the energy through your senses and anchor into your body as you do this. This is a great time to try anchoring into the environment by listening to the world around you, as described on page 189.

Connect to animals

Animals help us co-regulate. When they are healthy, their regulated nervous systems help our system get into the green zone. If you have a pet, or can spend time with an animal, focus on really being with them, looking in their eyes, stroking them, and cuddling them. Simply be around them, dropping in and out of connection if it feels too intense. Note: some pets have experienced trauma – rescue animals can sometimes have a trauma background, for example – but if you can connect with them, your nervous system can help theirs regulate too.

Connect to other people (while alone)

Reading or listening to audiobooks or podcasts are great ways to feel connected to people without needing to be physically in their presence. They allow you to empathise and be 'in the world' without leaving your home. Read or listen to people you want to connect with. Biographies and memoirs are great for this.

Connect to other people (for real)

Start slowly here by connecting with people who feel relatively neutral, and do this in places that feel safer. Even small daily interactions count and will signal safety to your nervous system. Take your time to slow down and look a cashier in the eye or smile at someone as you walk your dog. This may feel uncomfortable and that's okay – use the activation and anchoring techniques to help yourself regulate during these interactions. When you feel ready, aim for slightly longer interactions, remembering to stay focused on learning to help yourself feel safer as you do this.

Just like the soothing techniques, these ways of anchoring and connecting can signal safety to your nervous system and bring you into the ventral green zone. 'Can' is the operative word here because learning which techniques work is a process of trial and error. Because we all start from different places and with varying capacity, what works for one person won't necessarily work for another. Likewise, what helps you move into a sense of safety when you're starting from freeze mode is likely to be different from when you're in fight-flight mode.

Allowing and releasing

As we deepen our conversation with and connection to our body, we become increasingly able to notice and feel what's happening in it – noticing biological impulses, emotion and arousal energy. We also become willing and able to consciously *allow* these impulses, emotions and energy to complete and discharge. This is an important aspect of self-regulation, which we find becomes increasingly possible as we integrate all four capacities. In other words, as you're increasingly curious and aware, anchored into your wise adult self and feeling connected to your sense of agency, you'll find yourself increasingly able to listen, notice and allow biological impulses, emotion and trapped arousal energy to move through you.

One basic example of allowing a biological impulse to happen is noticing we need the toilet and then going. Or noticing that we're hot, so we take off a jumper. Or you might notice that your body is signalling to you that it's uncomfortable and in pain – you feel a twinge in your knee and sense that it needs to stretch, and you complete the biological impulse by stretching and moving your knee. It sounds simple, and in some ways it is, but many trauma survivors have learned to ignore and override their bodies' needs. Remember the main goal of what we're doing here is to help your body feel safer and more comfortable. Ignoring any biological impulse creates stress and tension – it keeps you in the orange or red zones.

I love the Somatic Experiencing (SE) practitioner Kimberly Ann Johnson's definition of trauma: trauma is stress without movement. This is because before, when we were younger, we wanted to act – to leave or fight – but we couldn't, so we froze. Our survival response didn't complete. To understand this, picture the huge flood of adrenaline and cortisol through our bodies as we experience fear and shock. Our mind and body are flooded with stress hormones to prepare us for action. But because the threat feels too big we can't mobilise the energy and move into action. So where does the energy go? Well, in many ways, it's still in our mind and body. It has morphed, and continues to morph, into anxiety, panic, overthinking and compulsions. Part of healing involves learning to healthily mobilise and release arousal energy from your system. We notice when arousal energy builds up and take action to allow it to move and discharge.

Every day, multiple times a day, we need to give ourselves the opportunity to allow and release this energy. There are many ways we can do this. It's a change in mindset. Instead of trying to manage, avoid or stop the fight-flight, freeze, fawn or collapse energy, we notice its presence and allow it to move through us in a safe way.

One example of this is noticing when you feel a flood of anger. Find a safe space and allow yourself to shout, make deep angry noises, stamp your feet and punch the air. Then allow smaller, more subtle energy release (like shaking your hands or rolling your head). This example makes it clear that as we talk about noticing and moving energy, we're also talking about noticing and moving emotion.

It's a really interesting process that involves conscious connection with your body, which is why this practice will feel easier as you move into greater conscious awareness and embodied safety. We stop being afraid of the energy and instead we mobilise and activate it in a small, safe way, then we allow it to discharge and taper out – almost like we're allowing our fight-flight energy and body to follow the bell curve. We allow it to move up, and then down, instead of not allowing it at all and pushing it back down.

I discussed this powerful allowing and releasing approach with Somatic Experiencing (SE) practitioner Sheryl Close. She highlighted the importance of titration (adjusting the 'dose') as we use these self-led tools:

> When engaging in allowing and releasing techniques, titration is essential. If an individual was to push themselves further than their capacity allows, they may experience overwhelm or shutdown. When you titrate a technique, you need to start slowly and gently. For example, if you are allowing and releasing sound, start quietly, giving space in between each sound and increasing the volume at a pace that feels manageable. Otherwise the internal movement and intensity may be too much, causing overwhelm, freeze, collapse or dissociation. Go slowly and take your time.

To bring more allowing and releasing into your day, it's helpful to just experiment with mindful movement and release. Stretching, stomping, dancing, yawning, sighing, crying and shouting can all bring release because they move energy in one way or another. If at any point it feels too much, stop and signal safety.

Here are some specific directions on how to move and release the different survival energies:

1. Stress energy (cortisol) wants to burn up. It wants you to hold difficult isometric contractions (such as chair pose or elbow plank) for as long as possible – do the exercise until you shake as it discharges.
2. Fight energy wants to use force. It wants you to stamp, hit a pillow or punching bag, shout or exhale loudly.
3. Flight energy wants to escape and find relief. It wants you to shake and hiss, as if you're letting out a pressure valve.

4. Freeze/fawn energy wants to escape and find relief but it also needs you to help it feel a little safer. It wants you to signal safety (for example by slowly circling your hips) and then release some of the arousal energy (try shaking or hissing).

5. Collapse energy wants to gently wake up. It needs you to move very slowly, like a flower unfurling. Try something as small as wiggling your toes or circling your wrists, or excuse yourself to the bathroom and wash your hands and/or face. Once you wake up, it wants you to help it release some arousal energy too.

A final note on connecting to your body safely

Like Naomi on page 173, we've all spent decades avoiding the body because it holds the emotions and wounding we want to push away. Our traumatic reactions disconnect us from our body in lots of different ways – dissociation, compulsive over-thinking and worrying are clear examples. Many behavioural adaptations, like compulsive busyness, also disconnect us from feeling. Using alcohol or food to numb out or get that fizzy adrenaline high are also behaviours that disconnect us from our body. Codependence – the habitual act of putting someone else's needs above our own – is also a way of discon-necting from ourselves. We anchor into someone else's experiences rather than our own. Scrolling endlessly through social media or numbing out watching TV are also common ways we disconnect from our body and emotions.

Reconnection to our body requires us to increasingly anchor our awareness physically. But as we drop into our body we *feel*, so it's not an easy process. Being more embodied requires us to support ourselves as we notice the feelings or beliefs that emerge as we drop into connection. This will come as you begin to integrate all four of the core capacities. Initially, to do this safely we only consciously connect to our body for short moments. If connection with your body, or any emotion or sensation, feels too intense, remember Principle Five: dip in and out of discomfort. So move your attention into your body, focusing on a sensation, emotion or body part, then allow your mind to wander or focus on something outside your body – for example, by noticing objects or sounds in the environment. In and out, in and out. We also practise noticing and naming any difficult emotions or sensations and then reassuring ourselves. For example: 'There's a lot of anxiety and tension in my chest. It's okay, everyone feels this way sometimes.'

As you play around with connection to your body, it's essential that you follow the Principles of Self-led Integration (page 156, if you need to refresh your memory). Every single one of them is relevant as you reconnect and will help you do this safely.

Chapter Seven

Capacity two: moving into presence, observation, curiosity and clarity

Previously we discussed the many ways you can signal safety to your nervous system and body using your imagination, touch, movement, different breath patterns, vibration, connection and release. Now we're going to talk about how you can move yourself into greater conscious awareness through presence, observation, curiosity and clarity. Increasing your capacity for awareness is an essential pillar of all healing and growth, because before we can create change in the direction we want and need, we must be able to *see* ourselves and our lives clearly.

In a myriad of different ways, I've been trying to help you see, feel and understand that in one way or another you've been on autopilot, sleepwalking and repeating old patterns without realising it. Trauma healing starts when something pierces our consciousness – we become aware of a problem. As we take action and move out of trauma-led patterns we increasingly move into conscious awareness and out of unconscious autopilot.

Greater conscious awareness of the trauma-led patterns we've been stuck in, and our authentic self that exists underneath these patterns, is the primary outcome we're trying to achieve. We achieve this increased awareness through presence, observation, curiosity and clarity. Integrating this capacity involves experiencing and playing around with the subtle differences between these different facets of awareness. Each state of awareness – presence, observation, curiosity and clarity – is experienced on a spectrum. At times we are fully in these states, whereas at other times we may only be partially in them. When we feel safe and regulated (in the green zone) we naturally flow in and out of each state of awareness. Here is a brief definition of these states:

Presence: this describes a state in which we're aware of the moment as it unfolds.[1] Our attention and awareness are anchored into the very moment we currently occupy – we are not preoccupied (as we are when we are worrying) or disconnected (as when we dissociate or feel self-conscious). At times we can be fully present and anchored into our body and environment; at other times we can also be somewhat present – for example we might be aware of our body and regulated, but with part of our attention on problem-solving a piece of work.

Observation: this is a subtle shift from presence into intentional non-judgemental listening and noticing. As with all these facets of awareness, we experience observation on a spectrum. At times, 100 per cent of our conscious awareness and attention can be observing.

When we're taking part in a conversation or making a cup of tea, just 5 per cent of our conscious awareness can be observing. This may sound a little abstract. Don't worry, I'm going to talk you through how to do this later in the chapter (see page 214).

Curiosity: this type of awareness is a slight shift from observation into open-minded listening and observing with the aim of understanding, rather than judging, concluding or winning. Curiosity is a natural facet of ventral vagal activation and regulation – the safer we feel, the more curious we can be.

Clarity: is experienced as we subtly shift once more from curiosity into understanding and instinctively knowing. Clarity is experienced as a sense that we can see ourselves and our lives as they truly are. It is a sense of anchored knowing and truth. We also become clear on the action, if any, we need to take. For this reason, clarity is an essential springboard into agency and self-led action. As we practise presence, observation and curiously observing, we move in and out of clarity.

Of all the capacities, the one described in this chapter – the capacity to move yourself into greater awareness through presence, observation, curiosity and clarity – is the one that has the most potential for instant gratification. And we all love that, don't we? I've noticed that for many of my clients, moving into greater awareness can bring almost instant relief. This makes sense to me. For those of us stuck in our minds, caught up in a barrage of old beliefs, parts and thoughts, learning to separate ourselves from these things can feel immediately divine.

We can test this theory now. Simply pause and connect to the present moment. Literally stop reading, moving, fidgeting, thinking, doing. Just pause and *be* where you are. Melt into the present moment, don't push or search. Now, consciously step back a little: observe yourself and the environment around you in a neutral way.

This may only feel good, or be possible, for a few seconds. If you feel yourself start to panic, simply put your hand on your heart, exhale and drop your shoulders and say to yourself, 'It's okay, you're safe' and come out of the practice.

This practice, which some refer to as a *sacred pause*, helps you experience presence and develop the capacity to observe without judgement. This kind of pause is more powerful than it may first appear because it helps build capacity while also interrupting trauma-led patterns. The moment you pause and melt into the present moment, you step out of old conditioning – you, quite literally, interrupt your trauma patterns. This also explains why it can feel uncomfortable – because we're diverting from our deeply ingrained neural map.

This sacred pause might remind you of the anchoring techniques in the previous chapter. You may have already started playing around with how to signal safety to your nervous system and body by anchoring into the present moment via your senses and your body. You may know the instant relief that comes from moving into presence and out of old patterns. All the capacities overlap, and anchoring is where capacities One and Two overlap. Presence can simultaneously signal safety *and* move us into greater awareness through observation.

Potentially, then, the primary difference between connecting to the present moment via our senses to signal safety and pausing and melting into the present moment to increase awareness is *intention*. As unremarkable as this sounds, it makes a difference to how we experience this kind of presence. When we use a pause to anchor and signal safety we do so to soothe and regulate. When we use a pause to move into awareness we do so to wake up, switch on our pre-frontal cortex and see with clarity. The *quality* of these practices is subtly different because of the intention behind them.

Integrating Capacity Two involves daily action. Every day, we practise increasing our awareness through presence, observation, curiosity and clarity. Slowly, we build the 'conscious awareness' muscle, training our mind to increasingly witness the present moment, ourselves and reality with curiosity so we can more clearly see ourselves and our lives. This involves intentional observation (for example, the intention to observe your thoughts). It's a gentle mix of increasingly moving into conscious awareness and intentionally directing your attention towards the patterns, parts of yourself, beliefs and truths you've been avoiding. First we increase our capacity to curiously witness the present moment, then we intentionally observe so we can see ourselves more clearly. In many ways, then, this capacity is the first step to greater authenticity and self-acceptance.

By the end of this chapter, you're going to understand how to harness your own power to move into presence, awareness and curiosity so you can observe yourself more honestly and clearly.

The Capacity Two Polarities

As I previously explained, polarities help us understand what we're moving from and to. They help us understand the difference between trauma and trauma healing, between the forest and the mountain top. The polarities that will help you better understand Capacity Two are:

- Preoccupied vs present
- Merged vs observing
- Closed mindedness vs openness
- Protective patterns vs expansiveness
- Fixed thinking vs curiosity
- Autopilot vs awareness
- Confusion vs clarity.

These polarities give you a sense of what the results of childhood trauma actually are (preoccupation, becoming enmeshed, closed-mindedness, protective patterns, fixed thinking/responses, being on autopilot). They also give you direction about where you're heading and what exists at the top of the mountain: presence, observation, openness, expansiveness, curiosity and greater awareness.

Self-led integration: A reminder

We integrate Capacity Two through daily action. It's helpful to think of this in two parts. First, we build our capacity to be more present, to witness and to be curious. We do this through longer daily practices, such as a daily meditation practice, and through a subtle change in how we approach each moment of the day. Second, we get intentionally curious about ourselves so we can move into greater awareness and clarity.

This chapter won't include a lot of tools, unlike the previous chapter. Integrating this capacity is a different process, and one I find clients are more comfortable with than the task of signalling safety. It also leads to insights and clarity, which in turn lead to a greater sense of agency, direction and control. Having said this, the process of moving into awareness is often painful. It doesn't feel safe to see and feel all the things we've been subconsciously avoiding for years. For this reason, we have no choice but to take it slow. We can only integrate this capacity if we're simultaneously integrating the other three. To see and feel *reality* in a safe way that leads to healing, we must also be increasingly signalling safety to our nervous system and body, connecting to our adult self, and taking self-led action in our lives. This is why we follow the Principles of Self-led Integration – they ensure all four capacities are developing simultaneously no matter where we are in our healing journey.

In particular, as you practise Capacity Two, please remember principles One, Four, Five, Seven and Eleven:

- Principle One: Stretch don't stress – 1 per cent more is enough.
- Principle Four: Dip into discomfort – pendulate into and out of uncomfortable awareness.
- Principle Five: Find your way back to green (this is your north star).
- Principle Seven: Respond with adult compassion.
- Principle Eleven: Find soft places to land.

To safely build this capacity, we move into conscious awareness slowly and gently – 1 per cent more each day is enough (Principle One). As you move into awareness, you will feel and observe things that are uncomfortable. Notice if you're afraid of the discomfort and signal safety to hold yourself through it – experiencing it is part of increasing our window of tolerance. But likewise, aim to dip into and out of it (Principle Three). Do this by moving from discomfort into the green zone (Principle Four). Practise holding yourself through any moments of discomfort in a new, compassionate way. You do not need to shower yourself with loving affirmations (although it would be lovely if you did). But you do need to aim to respond with a little more kindness, care and adult reason (Principle Seven). Responding from this place, as a wise, loving adult, is the work of integrating Capacity Three, which I'll cover in the next chapter. But you can start now by responding with adult compassion as you journey into greater awareness.

Finally, moving into awareness can feel overwhelming, so we need to be able to process what we discover – we need a soft place to land. Journalling is essential as you move through the second part of this capacity; I have described the practice of journalling in more detail on page 226, but essentially, this means writing down your thoughts and feelings using pen and paper. However, this may not be enough. If you feel overwhelmed, scattered and confused, or if you simply yearn for another human to be in the spaghetti with you, find people and spaces that can hold you (Principle Eleven).

From tomorrow, to begin to integrate Capacity Two, aim to use a deeper practice daily (for instance, try a two-minute meditation practice) and just one of the conscious living practices daily – say, pausing and becoming present moment-by-moment. Build your capacity for presence, observation, curiosity and awareness before you move into intentional observation of your trauma-led patterns.

Awareness as self

As we move through the four capacities of trauma healing, we build on and expand your sense of self. In Capacity One, I used the term 'self' as synonymous with ventral vagal activation and regulation. Here in Capacity Two, regulation is still the foundation of self, but we also come to understand self as a facet of awareness that exists when we're in, or moving towards, regulation.

Here, self is your seat of conscious awareness. It's the subtle shift of awareness that happens as you move back ever so slightly to observe yourself. It's us observing ourselves and the world around us. It's us witnessing without judgement. I love the spiritual teacher Ram Dass's quote: '*The witness coexists alongside your normal consciousness as another layer of awareness, as the part of you that is awakening.*'[2]

The tools and practices in this chapter are designed to help you experience your self as this higher consciousness, witness and observer. To help you pull back and create a gap between you and the autopilot you've been stuck in.

Experiencing self in this way is not just about seeing ourselves with more adult perspective and neutrality. It's also a powerful form of centring and regulating. Self as your seat of conscious awareness brings an energy and a curious presence that anchors and soothes.

Safety first

The practices described in this chapter are intentionally designed to develop and deepen Capacity Two, but the process of moving into conscious awareness starts as we begin to signal safety to our nervous systems. The mind struggles to settle into the present moment if the body feels unsafe. All self-led action we take to bring ease and comfort to the body and move out of survival helps the mind move out of protective unconscious autopilot and into expansive conscious awareness. Bear this in mind as you begin to integrate Capacity Two.

A familiar example of this is how painfully hard it is to meditate if we're anxious. In this oh-so common example, we first need to notice that there's too much arousal energy in our body for us to settle into presence. Noticing leads to the next step: realising that before we meditate, we need to take action to signal safety. First, we could first discharge some of the energy through an isometric contraction (like an elbow plank – see page 196). Then we could use a soothing breath count (such as polyvagal breathing – see page 185) to activate the ventral vagal nerve. This self-led action creates more embodied safety, which facilitates presence. As we notice there's been a small shift in our physiology – perhaps slightly less contraction and tension in the chest, or a feeling of lightness – we can then move more comfortably into a meditation practice.

I used this example because although it's extremely common, clients often overlook it because they struggle to notice the anxiety and force themselves into a painful meditation practice. This makes sense because we're used to functioning with extremely high levels of anxiety – pushing through in survival is the norm. As you're starting to use these daily practices, check in with your body before you begin. If you notice a lot of survival energy, take some time to create a little more embodied safety by using the soothing, anchoring, connecting or releasing techniques from Capacity One before you try to settle into presence.

Remember this too if, as you're curiously observing, you begin to move into survival (for example, you might notice you feel more anxious). This is also an extremely common experience. Don't just push through. Pause and use the Capacity One tools to move back into the green zone, then move back into awareness (Principle Three – dip into and out of discomfort, and Principle Five – move back into green).

Daily practices to increase awareness

Before we can intentionally see and feel our trauma-led patterns, we need to increase our capacity for awareness. Here I'm going to describe three types of practice that are proven to move us into greater conscious awareness:

- Meditation
- Yoga nidra and non-sleep deep rest (NSDR)
- Mindfulness.

These practices are reliable, evidence-based ways to increase your conscious awareness, and therefore, your capacity to witness and be curious. Like everything in this book, neuroplasticity is the power behind these positive, expansive changes. Meditation, yoga nidra and mindfulness have been studied extensively, so we're building a clear picture of how they harness neuroplasticity and positively impact the physical structure of the brain to permanently alter our capacity for conscious awareness (presence, observing, curiosity and clarity).

One of the most fascinating discoveries from neuroscience research is that meditation increases our capacity for awareness by radically interrupting the survival response at a neural level. To understand why interrupting survival brings us into greater awareness we have to remember our polarities. When we're in survival (the orange and red zones) we're in patterns of disconnection and autopilot, rather than connection and awareness. Awareness is naturally available to us when we're in the green zone, so 'radically interrupting the survival response' at a neural level will in turn increase our capacity for presence, observation and curiosity.

Research has consistently demonstrated that the amygdala, an almond-shaped, paired structure in our brain responsible for triggering the survival response by noticing threat, is smaller in meditators than non-meditators.[3] Although more research is needed, altered hippocampal dimensions (that is, changing the shape and size of a region of the brain) may be one result of meditation-induced stress reduction. The hippocampus is a region known to function as a brake that curbs the release of stress hormones.[4] This has the potential to help us experience more embodied safety, as well as to move us into greater awareness.

Research into how meditation affects brainwaves also demonstrates why and how a daily meditation practice increases our capacity for awareness. This research is also incredibly intriguing. There are five main types of brain waves: alpha, beta, delta, theta and gamma. Alpha brain waves sit in the centre of the brain wave hierarchy. We experience them when we're aware and awake but also relaxed and regulated. Studies have shown that meditation increases alpha wave activity in the brain, even beyond the meditation itself.[5] This state of awareness – aware, awake and regulated – is precisely what we're hoping to develop as we integrate this capacity. This research makes it clear that meditation is a sure-fire way to build this muscle.

Yoga nidra is an ancient deep relaxation practice that blends meditation and guided visualisation. It's a state of conscious rest that allows the body to relax while the mind remains alert and aware.[6] It's similar to meditation, but uses our imagination and our attention to increase regulation and activate the ventral vagal nerve. In 2022, Dr Andrew Huberman coined the term non-sleep deep rest (NSDR) to describe practices that 'guide your brain and body into a state of deep relaxation without falling asleep completely'.[7] Huberman's NSDR is very similar to yoga nidra. They just have slightly different flavours, with yoga nidra using more traditional yogic language and imagery and NSDR using the language and imagery of the nervous system.

Some really interesting research conducted in 2011 observed the impact of yoga nidra on veterans with combat-induced PTSD. Practising yoga nidra significantly increased the veterans' feelings of self-awareness, relaxation, peace and self-efficacy, and reduced their rage, anxiety and emotional reactivity.[8] This research is highly supportive of incorporating yoga nidra into our daily routine as we move through trauma healing.

Lastly, let me tell you about mindfulness. Mindfulness is the practice of paying attention to the present moment without judgement and being fully aware of where we are and what we're doing. If you're doing a double take (or yawning), I understand – it's been talked about a lot over the years. Mindfulness simply describes presence and observation. Mindfulness as a concept has its roots in Buddhist philosophy, and as a practice took off around the world in the 1960s and 70s. I'm using it here because although it's hard for me to find research on 'presence and observation', mindfulness has been extensively practised and studied. I also think it's helpful for you to understand the overlap of all these terms.

Some of the most compelling mindfulness research demonstrates that mindfulness training (a combination of mindfulness meditation practices and psycho-education) leads to greater sustained attention, working memory and presence in everyday life, as well as feeling less preoccupied, and experiencing less worry and rumination.[9]

Okay, I'm going to stop throwing research studies at you. I hope something caught your attention and convinced you that a daily practice of meditation, yoga nidra, NSDR and/or mindfulness will greatly (greatly!) increase your capacity for awareness and support your self-led trauma healing journey.

Choose one of the practices, and from tomorrow, aim to do it daily. You can find information about further resources, such as guides and audios that will help you start experimenting with these four awareness practices, in Appendix C.

Conscious living

As well as the longer daily practices, building Capacity Two requires us to approach how we relate to our day differently. We aim to increasingly live with more awareness – more presence, observation and curiosity – which in turn leads to a greater sense of clarity. This starts as a daily intention to practise this new way of relating throughout the day. For some, it feels the most natural to practise this as a *response*: as we notice we're once again lost in worry, say, we take self-led action to gently move back into awareness and out of autopilot. For others, it feels easiest to practise this in a more structured way: as we plan our day, we schedule in time for presence, observation and curiosity. Neither approach is better – they both serve to increase our capacity for awareness.

Remember that it's wildly unrealistic to expect yourself to move from autopilot into conscious living quickly. In fact, taking an extreme approach will potentially harm and trigger you. Go gently as you reach for, and play with, awareness. One per cent more awareness tomorrow really is good enough.

It's also essential to remember that signalling safety through soothing, anchoring, connecting or releasing is often necessary before, during or after you try to settle into the present moment.

Conscious living as a response

As you go through the day, aim to notice when you feel particularly swamped by, and lost in, your thoughts or emotions – a sense of having disconnected from the present moment and your body. First, take action to soothe, anchor, connect or release. This doesn't have to take long – just provide a little more safety before you move back into the present moment. Next, pause and move into presence, observation and/or curious observation using the guides below.

Conscious living as a structured practice

As you start your day, schedule in time for presence, observation and curiosity. Thirty seconds is enough – this isn't about carving out huge amounts of time. Little and often is what we're going for. Phone reminders work well – you could set a reminder on the hour to pause. For those who dislike phone reminders, instead you can commit to pausing during every transition – say, before you start work, after you have lunch and so on.

When the timer goes off, or it's the allocated time, first take action to soothe, anchor, connect or release. Next, pause and move into presence, observation and/or curious observation using the guides below.

Presence

To move into presence, simply pause and move into connection with the present moment using your senses and awareness. This is about consciously controlling your attention and focus. Listen to the sounds around you, look around you with a gentle gaze or anchor into your body – focus your attention on your breath or another body part that feels safe. As I described previously, it may only feel comfortable to do this for a few seconds. If it feels uncomfortable, use a tool to signal safety to your nervous system (see page 165) and then, if it feels okay to, move back into present moment connection. This pendulation will keep you safe and help you build capacity.

Observation: What am I experiencing right now?

To move into observation, we observe ourselves in a *neutral* way. Every human is capable of observing their own thoughts and experience – this skill is part of what makes us human. To do this, pause and ask yourself this simple question: 'What am I experiencing and feeling right now?'

Consciously step back a little so you can observe your body, mind, emotions and behaviour in a more detached way. Slowly, and with as much neutrality (separation and regulation) as you can, notice and name your experience – your behaviours, emotions, sensations and thoughts. The acronym BEST (behaviours, emotions, sensations, thoughts) can help you remember what you're aiming to observe, but ignore this if it feels too prescriptive. We're observing and describing without judging or changing. This could sound like:

- 'There's a lot of anxiety in my body – my heart is beating fast and my mind is scattered.'
- 'I'm exhausted – I feel my eyes wanting to shut.'
- 'My mind feels confused and foggy.'
- 'I have a sinking feeling in my stomach.'
- 'I feel content and warm.'
- 'I feel sad and want to cry.'
- 'My arms feel tingly and hot.'
- 'My mind is whirring with thoughts about work.'
- 'My chest is constricted and there's a heavy feeling – it's hard to breathe.'

Some find it more calming to use one-word labelling, to help them stay present and in body-connection and not get pulled into overthinking. This could sound like:

- 'Anxiety'
- 'Scattered'
- 'Stomach'
- 'Sad'
- 'Preoccupied'
- 'Grumpy'
- 'Tension.'

Remember to only stay with an observation/feeling for a short moment. Feel/see it, but then take action to soothe and signal safety.

Curiosity

We move into curiosity as we become open and interested in our own experience and the experience of those around us. We're curious when we aim to understand rather than judge, conclude or win. Because we aim to understand, our observations are agenda-free and gentle, so they lead to flow, connection and regulation (rather than rigidity, conflict and dysregulation). It's a feeling state, not a thought process, so I can't give you a script. But remember you can seamlessly move from presence and observation into curiosity by shifting into open-hearted interest and wonder. To do this, pause and ask yourself this simple, curious question: '*I wonder* what I'm experiencing and feeling right now?'

In response to this question, you can pull in even more curiosity by answering it with more questions, interest and wonder. Questions naturally pull in more curiosity, but asking *how* or *what* questions rather than *why* questions tends to lead to greater regulated curiosity, because they move us towards our experience rather than back into the cognitive mind. Remember that the curiosity itself will move you towards the green zone. This could sound like:

- 'There's tension in my body today – that's really interesting, I wonder how I can create a little ease.'
- 'Wow, I really feel like I want to give up today – I'm curious about that; I wonder what that relates to?'
- 'Joe's being curt and grumpy today – that's interesting!'
- 'I can't stop eating today – that's interesting. I wonder what's going on?'
- 'I'm so adrenalised today – interesting!'
- 'I feel like such a failure today – I wonder what this is about?'

Remember that the goal of curiosity isn't to find an answer – it's to help ease tension, switch on neuroplasticity, anchor us back into self and create a sense of separation from our trauma and old patterning. Curiosity is an open-minded energy – we're interested in something rather than judging it. The prompts above are just there to give you a sense of what I mean. In practice, curiosity is a feeling, not a script. At the highest level, exploring curiosity means getting curious about what curiosity actually feels like! How does it feel to be curious? Spending some time exploring and feeling into this question is likely to be more beneficial than just using the prompts above.

Into action

Every day, multiple times a day, aim to move into presence, observation or the energy of curiosity. This practice will get easier and feel more natural the more you use it. At times, you may find that moving into these facets of awareness is enough to move you out of an old trauma-led pattern and into regulation and self-connection. In its simplicity and effectiveness, awareness is one of the most powerful self-led tools you have at your disposal.

Clarity

Clarity isn't something you can practise. It's an outcome, not a daily exercise. Having said this, there are a few things you can do (over and above practising presence, observation and curiosity) to assist clarity. First, don't panic if you feel confused (which you will, a lot). Confusion is a common experience for those with childhood trauma. Weirdly, we can facilitate clarity by accepting our confusion, uncertainty and not knowing instead of responding with judgement or panic. This is because clarity comes naturally as a result of regulation and self-connection. Anything that pulls us back into survival mode will move us away from, not towards, clarity. Here, then, we facilitate clarity by allowing and accepting times when we have none. This could sound like:

- 'I feel confused. That's okay, it will all become clear over time.'
- 'I trust that I'll understand when I need to.'
- 'My body will show me what I need to know, when I need to know it.'
- 'I don't know, and that's okay.'
- 'I don't have to figure all this out.'

These simple statements can move us into regulation, self-connection, and ultimately, clarity, because they help us let go, soothe and reassure. Give them a try if and when you feel confused as you're doing this observation work.

When to move into intentional observation

Once you sense that you've started to integrate this practice, move into intentional observation of your trauma patterns. Signs you have started to integrate the awareness practice are:

- You feel less resistance to moving into presence, observation and curiosity.
- You can easily pause and move into presence, observation and curiosity when you are not dysregulated.
- You can pause and move into presence, observation and curiosity when you are dysregulated.

- You can pause and move into presence, observation and curiosity when you are experiencing a triggered reaction.

Don't wait for perfection – you don't have to be able to perfectly and consistently move into presence, observation and curiosity. But likewise, don't be in a rush to move into intentional observation. Allow this capacity to build before you dive into the deeper work.

Moving into awareness

Before we move into the intentional observation work, I want to tell you about a client of mine. Maddie is 31 years old. She lives alone in Geneva, where she works for an international bank. The best way to describe Maddie is highly strung. But she's also got it all. Maddie has an incredible life – she has a beautiful apartment and luxury clothes, and travels extensively as part of her job. Maddie made her way to me via a referral. A friend of hers lovingly suggested that perhaps all the work and stress and 'perfecting' wasn't serving her – that perhaps Maddie wanted and needed something a little gentler.

On the one hand, Maddie knows all is not well. She's highly stressed and anxious. She also has a brutal exercise regimen and an extremely restrictive diet. Occasionally she purges food a compulsive behaviour that started when she was a teen at boarding school. But on the other hand, Maddie is aware that she's extremely successful and the success provides her with self-esteem. The success works against her acknowledging her wounding. I'm sure you can hear that this juxtaposition (which is very common in those with unresolved childhood trauma) prevents healing because it's so easy for us to move back into denial and autopilot. There's wounding, pain and trauma, but we've also adapted to protect ourselves, structuring our lives in a way that 'proves' there is nothing wrong.

Healing childhood trauma requires greater awareness. It requires us to look at our choices, emotions, thoughts and behaviours with greater curiosity. It also requires greater willingness to acknowledge our problems, pain and patterning. Initially, this curious observation and increased awareness wasn't an option for Maddie because she didn't have enough regulation and embodied safety. Before she was able to see, she needed to feel just a little safer.

For the first three months, I helped Maddie stabilise and self-regulate. Maddie really took to it – she enjoyed the physiological approach to trauma healing and happily practised the Capacity One tools and techniques. Towards the end of the three months, Maddie started a daily yoga nidra practice, then she created a short morning meditation for herself.

Initially Maddie came to sessions activated, distracted and stressed. She struggled to settle into the session. After four months, Maddie was calmer and a little more present when she came to sessions. Because Maddie was better able to self-regulate and was increasing her capacity for conscious awareness through yoga nidra and meditation, she became increasingly able to curiously observe (be in) reality. Maddie's observations and our conversations became more and more honest as she moved into genuine curiosity about what she was experiencing. As we moved through this work she was able to talk about her experiences with a little more neutrality and space.

I'm telling you about Maddie because her journey through

trauma healing illustrates that curiosity and awareness are fuelled by regulation and safety. You can't force yourself into seeing and knowing. It has to flow. And it will only flow if you build capacity slowly and steadily, and make Capacity One the foundation of your journey. As you move into intentional observation, or practise conscious living, you may feel strong triggered protective reactions pulling you away from this work and back into autopilot. Know that this okay and common. And when this happens, take it as a sign that your nervous system is asking for more safety and regulation (soothing, anchoring and connection). If you can't achieve the regulation you need alone, consider working with a practitioner to help you create enough safety and stability in your system to allow the work to progress.

Intentional observation

Intentional observation is about observing our triggered survival response with the intention of seeing and understanding the trauma-led patterns we're stuck in. Intentional observation and the questions we curiously ask about these observations help us begin to process (understand, move and assimilate) our trauma. This happens as we untangle the spaghetti – teasing apart our reaction – while in connection with our adult self, allowing us to make connections and finding meaning in a new way. It brings an adult perspective to our experience and reactions, and the new understanding we find helps us process and move out of autopilot.

We begin to process and make sense of our experience and patterning as we observe them during the day in a new way – by signalling safety and intentionally moving into presence,

221

observation and curiosity. This *new way* of observing ourselves during the day is the foundation of what we're doing here. But, we also achieve this retrospectively through journalling, particularly when we do this in a structured way – remaining anchored into our regulated adult self while answering specific questions that call us to look at different aspects of ourselves and our trauma patterning.

Untangling your survival response

Your survival response shows up in your mind as thought patterns and mental states, in your body as sensations and physiological symptoms, as emotions, and as behaviours. As you started to integrate Capacity One, you started to notice and respond (signal safety) when you felt yourself move into survival. So there's really nothing new here, we're just doing what you're already doing with a little more presence and curiosity, so you can begin to get clarity on your most common survival patterns.

These patterns consist of an external trigger, such as conflict, or an internal trigger like a pain in our leg or a thought, that reminds us of our past and activates an old wounding (an old emotion or belief). Because we feel unsafe we move up into survival – into fight, flight, freeze, fawn or collapse – and into a protective, old response pattern. This pattern starts in the nervous system as our amygdala picks up a threat. We experience survival in our body, mind, emotions and behaviour.

We need to untangle our triggered survival response because it holds really useful information about our trauma and what we need to do to heal. As you move through this work, you'll become more aware of the old wounding, emotions and beliefs that are triggered by current situations in adult life. Seeing this old *stuff* clearly, and with an adult perspective, is the first step to reclaiming our agency and being able to hold ourselves through these moments rather than reacting to or from them.

The mind

Trauma affects how we think and what we think about. It's remarkable how common the main trauma-led thought patterns are. These are ways that our wounding and our protective adaptations (the many ways we learn to cope with the wounding) show up in our mind and thinking. These states of mind and ways of thinking can be triggered subconsciously when our nervous system picks up on a threat. They correlate with fight (which can show up as irritability or defensiveness), flight (which can manifest as an urgency to plan or ruminating on fears), freeze (in the form of procrastination, worry or confusion), fawn (which shows up as feelings of insecurity and a fixation on others), and collapse (which mentally manifests as despair or giving up). See Appendix D for a fuller list of how survival shows up in our minds.

Behaviours

As you'd expect, observing our behaviours tends to be easier than observing our minds. Appendix D also includes a list of behaviours that commonly indicate that our wounding and survival response has been triggered. These behaviours tend to be compulsive – we feel a compelling urge to do them. We're also interested in patterns of behaviour over the day and the absence of behaviours (things we know we need to do but don't follow through on). Anything that feels driven by an urge is noteworthy.

Emotions and sensations

Observing this aspect of our trauma wounding and the survival response it triggers can be the most challenging to see and separate from. This makes sense because the mind and compulsive behaviours are where we hide from the body and the emotion it holds. Observing mind and behaviours with more neutrality, detachment and curiosity is hard. Observing feelings with the same curious energy is even harder because we're aiming to see, feel and be interested in the thing we've been avoiding. Although it's true that it's harder, it's also true that when you practise Principle Four (dipping in and out of uncomfortable emotions, page 158) you're observing your feelings. Likewise, when you self-regulate (noticing and responding, pages 169–72), you're observing your feelings. During the observation work (page 214), you were observing your feelings. You're already integrating the capacity to safely observe, experience and be with your feelings. Here, we're just taking this to the next level by consciously linking your emotions to your sensations, and getting curious about how your feelings are part of a broader response pattern.

You can find a fuller list of emotions and sensations in Appendix D. It's common to experience more than one emotion/sensation at a time. Becoming aware of all the emotions and sensations that are present, and the contradictions between them, is part of what we're trying to do. It's perfectly possible to feel both excited and afraid, or hopeful and despairing, say.

Please be mindful that emotions are energy and sensations in the body so they can morph and change as we observe them. Noticing how you experience emotions and survival responses in your body is a big part of trauma healing. It's also a weird new thing. Try to notice and get curious about emotions and sensations in your body, but also know that this is very hard. It's even harder if you're stressed or strung out. To safely, curiously observe your emotions and sensations, you're likely to need to signal safety more often and/ or acknowledge when doing this work feels too much (and therefore *not* do it!). Signalling safety really does have to come first – it's the doorway to being able to move into presence, observation and curiosity. If you struggle to get any sense of what you're feeling, take it as a sign that more regulation is needed.

Beliefs

Traumatic beliefs are the conclusions we came to about ourselves, others or the world during the initial traumatic experience. These kinds of beliefs drive the triggered reaction we experience in adult life and sit at the heart of our trauma patterning. In many ways, they are our trauma.

Over time, traumatic beliefs (such as I'm bad, I'm disgusting, I'm worthless, I'm getting it all wrong, other people can't be trusted or the world is unsafe) weave their way into our thinking and identity. They shape the way we relate to ourselves, others and the world. They determine our expectations, relationships and life choices. They prevent us from healing and changing – they are pernicious and highly damaging. Bringing these kinds of beliefs into conscious awareness and learning how to see and separate from them, then, is an essential part of trauma healing. In Appendix D you can also find a fuller list of traumatic beliefs.

Observing the survival response

There are a couple of different approaches you can take to observing your survival response day-to-day.

Option one: in real-time
The first is to make notes in your journal as you move through the day, noticing whenever you've moved into survival. Briefly jot down what you're noticing about your reaction. Include what the trigger was, and whatever you can observe going on in your mind, body, emotions and/or behaviour.

Option two: at the end of the day
Or, rather than making notes in real time, towards the end of each day, grab your journal and answer this question: 'I wonder when and how I moved into survival today?' Use the information in Appendix D, to help.

Journalling

At the end of the day, choose one aspect of your survival response and answer the questions below. Focus on an aspect of your response that you're genuinely curious about – a part of your thinking, behaviour, beliefs, symptoms, emotions or sensations that you want to better understand. Answer as many or as few questions as you want:

• I wonder what triggered this protective survival response?
• I wonder why this trigger feels so threatening to me?

- I wonder which thoughts, behaviours, sensations, symptoms and emotions accompany this reaction?
- I wonder whether this reaction is part of fight, flight, freeze, fawn or collapse (or a mixture of two states)? Refer to Diagram 4, page 172 if you're unsure.
- I wonder what old emotion and/or belief is driving this protective reaction?
- I wonder what this protective reaction is trying to protect me from? It can help to frame this as, 'I wonder what its best intention is for me?'
- I wonder what the younger part of me that's reacting needs from adult me to help it feel safer?
- I wonder how familiar this reaction is? How long have I carried this fear/belief and been reacting this way to try to cope?

As you journal, please approach your observations and writing with curiosity and compassion. This is particularly necessary to ensure you don't move into overthinking or a strong triggered reaction. To help ensure the journalling process is compassionate and anchored, please:

- Regulate first, using the Capacity One tools.
- Write concisely, using clear, straightforward langugage whenever you can, to ensure you remain clear and in your observer self. Consider using bullet-points if it helps you remain grounded.
- Focus on one aspect of your trauma patterning at a time, be mindful of avoiding overwhelm by keeping journalling sessions short and focused.

- Take days off journalling – you're likely to lose motivation and perspective if you do this daily without any breaks. Trauma healing requires time out from trauma healing.

Structured journalling – answering questions with the aim of unblending from our trauma and increasing our adult perspective – is very different from stream-of-consciousness journalling. The purpose here is to remain in our compassionate observer self by answering specific questions. But if you wish, and find it cathartic, also use stream-of-consciousness journalling – writing freehand, allowing the words and emotion to flow without any need to find out more or 'be an adult', aiming only to allow yourself to release emotion and intensity.

The dance

If you've already started practising greater awareness, you may understand what I mean when I say that integrating this capacity involves moving between safety, awareness and survival.

The safer we feel, the more awareness and reality we can open to. This awareness, though, initially feels unsafe, so we move back into survival. We aim to move into awareness of survival by noticing it, and then take action to move back into safety, so we can then move back into awareness – and so it goes on. We move backwards and forwards, and as we do, we build capacity and widen our window of tolerance. Understanding that this process is okay, ideal even, is critical to keep us feeling motivated and safe as we increase awareness. Parts of you may get triggered as you notice you've moved back into survival – for example, judging the anxiety you're experiencing as bad, wrong or a sign you're unwell. Try to become aware of these reactions, and take time to respond with compassion (Principle Seven).

This is the dance of trauma healing, providing you dip in and out and signal safety. Go slowly and take your time – slow is fast in trauma healing.

Chapter Eight

Capacity three: receiving yourself with perspective and compassion

Integrating Capacity Three is, in my humble opinion, an expansive, empowering journey. Everything in this book is designed to create contrast, because *difference* is necessary to interrupt old trauma-led patterns and move out of auto-pilot. But the Capacity Three ways of being, relating and responding feel more than *different*. For most, experiencing Capacity Three – receiving yourself with adult perspective and compassion – feels radically new. For most, actually, it's the nearest we come to understanding in real time what trauma healing truly feels like.

As we develop this capacity, we start to view our trauma-led survival adaptations as younger parts of our psyche. For example, we might look at our anxiety as an anxious *part* of ourselves, rather than our whole self. As we take self-led action to see and separate from these *parts*, we reconnect back to our adult self and experience a sense of relief, and over time, stabilisation. As we go one step further and receive these protective, wounded *parts* of our being with compassion, as a wise, loving adult, we experience a new sense of internal settling and ease. As we move into deeper self-led healing work with these parts, we experience a powerful sense of resolution and release.

This capacity, then, takes things a step further than the work we've been doing up to now. We're moving from building capacities that impact measurable aspects of our body, such as our nervous system, and mind, like our presence, curiosity and awareness, to building a capacity that impacts something deeper and wholly intangible: the psyche and sense of self.

Trauma affects the body and mind. It affects our behaviour and relationships. But it also deeply affects our sense of self – our perception of the characteristics, traits, abilities and beliefs that define us. Not only does it predispose us to developing a negative, shame-based sense of self, it also affects our capacity to develop a sense of self at all. Many with unresolved child-hood trauma feel as if they're disconnected from who they truly are – that how they present, react and show up is out of alignment somehow.

There are many reasons childhood trauma leads to this self-disconnection. Here, I want to help you get a sense of just how damaging a lack of support is for a child's develop-ing sense of self and internal experience. Children internalise whatever support model they receive in childhood. If they receive good enough levels of support, they internalise them, and become able to support themselves later in life. In response to their parents' patience, reason, compassion and validation, they develop these qualities within themselves. Without even realising it, children in these homes naturally become their own support system. They can be patient and compassion-ate with themselves. They can see the bigger picture and be their own voice of reason. They can validate their own experience and accept every part of themselves. As a result, they feel safe enough to operate authentically as they move through the world.

As we imagine what the inner world of someone *without* childhood trauma might look like, we can visualise a strong, whole, loving self at the centre. This anchoring self acts as a wise, loving adult to guide, soothe and keep things in perspective. It is their ballast and anchor-point, creating regulation and balance internally, and alignment externally.

This supportive, reasonable, internalised adult is largely absent from the day-to-day inner world of those with unresolved childhood trauma. Because we have no internalised source of support and anchoring, we develop extreme adaptations (*parts*) to help us cope and survive. In place of an anchoring adult is, say, a taskmaster part or an anxious part, trying to motivate us through fear. Reinstating an anchoring adult into our inner world is essential if we wish to heal childhood trauma.

Therapeutically, then, we can't fully explain trauma healing without talking about the intangible magical aspects of being human – our psyche, spirit or sense of self. For this reason, nervous system approaches that do not also address these can only take us so far. Regulation is the foundation, but from here, we need to move into the intangible realm of *self*.

Deep therapeutic work that helps us explore our psyche and sense of self is often undertaken with a psychotherapist – this is their MO. A psychotherapist is trained in the skilful, safe exploration of the human psyche. If you wish, and when you're ready, you too can move into collaborative healing work with a trauma-trained therapist. But it's also true that your sense of self and psyche are *yours*. *You* can learn to take self-led action to safely explore your inner world, begin to reinstate an internal anchoring adult and bring greater relief, settling and resolution. *You* can create deep healing within your sense of self.

The parts approach

A parts approach is a way of understanding your mind and your self-concept – your idea of who you are. It's also a technique that's often used by psychotherapists, psychologists, somatic practitioners (that is, people who work with the body) and coaches. Most importantly, it's a technique you can develop to heal yourself. Parts psychology isn't new, but we're all talking about it a lot more because it's such a helpful model for understanding and healing childhood trauma. So, parts work is a psychological model of the self *and* it's a powerful healing methodology.

Parts work is based on the concept that within each of us there are many different parts, or personalities. This isn't a new idea. Carl Jung brought the term *inner child* into mainstream psychology over a century ago. Inner child work is an example of a parts approach. The concept of an *inner critic* has also become mainstream. The widespread use of these two concepts highlights how natural and easy it feels to view ourselves and our personality as consisting of different parts with different roles.

Whether we have unresolved childhood trauma or not, we all have different parts that reflect different aspects of our personality, our roles in life and our preferences. Think about how many times you've heard someone say something like: 'Part of me wants to quit and run and tell everyone to go to hell, but the rational part of me knows that I need to stay and figure out a way through.' Or: 'Part of me knows I'm doing really well, but another part tells me I'm screwing everything up.'

The Internal Family Systems (IFS) model of parts work is comprehensive and instinctive, and for that reason is becoming a leading therapeutic model for working with childhood trauma. Richard Schwartz, who founded IFS, explains that 'parts' are natural – they're not the product of trauma. They're a normal facet of the human psyche. But for some, trauma and attachment injuries – damage to the bond we have with our primary care givers – move our parts into roles that can be destructive. Schwartz writes: 'A lot of the time these parts don't know that you've grown up. They're "frozen" in the time of the trauma and keep doing whatever extreme things they did to protect you when you were young.'[1]

Think about any survival adaptation that started during your childhood – maybe overthinking, striving, anxiety, procrastination, compulsive overeating, people-pleasing – well, within parts work, we get curious about the part of us that acts out the adaptation.

Instead of stating, 'I'm a people-pleaser', we move into parts work as we more truthfully say, 'Part of me wants to people-please.' This simple statement separates us slightly from the part, and in doing so, helps us reconnect back to our self – the anchoring adult that exists underneath all the parts and adaptations. Most likely, alongside a 'people-pleasing part', there's also a part that's had enough of putting everyone else before ourselves. The people-pleasing part can feel so intense and all-encompassing that we struggle to hear the whisper of another part saying,

'I've had enough', and beneath that, a younger, wounded part saying, 'I'm getting it all wrong.' As we see and validate the parts that are activated, we more deeply understand ourselves and reconnect back to our adult self – the 'I' that exists underneath the wounding and the survival adaptations.

Can you feel the shift we're starting to make? As you integrated capacities One and Two, we talked about your trauma-led thoughts, sensations, emotions and behaviours. Now, as we integrate Capacity Three, everything we experience outside of self is understood as a *part*. This is a big change in how we're communicating about trauma, so don't worry if you don't fully *get it*. You don't have to perfectly understand the idea of parts. Allow the idea to flow over you. Sit with it. Allow it to *percolate* (as one of my wonderful clients once said) and try to trust that this idea will come alive as you start to practise it.

In this book I talk about two *types* of part – the parts that hold the initial wounding and the parts that are trying to protect us from it:

1. Wounded younger parts that experienced the original trauma: the parts of you that carry the traumatic beliefs and emotions, and have the memory of the trauma.
2. Protective parts that adapted so they could keep you safe, and cope with life and the wounding.

Wounded younger parts are vulnerable. They carry intense emotions like fear, anger, abandonment, sadness, despair or terror. They also carry traumatic beliefs that were created during their traumatic experience, such as 'I'm unlovable,' 'I'm bad,' 'I'm too much,' 'I'm getting it all wrong,' or 'People aren't safe.'

Examples of common wounded parts are:

235

- As a young part of us that feels abandoned and unlovable.
- As a part that feels isolated and separate, believing they don't belong and can't connect to others.
- As a part that feels powerless and out of control.
- As a part of us that feels 'too much', believing they are too much for other people to handle or love.
- As a part that feels 'not enough', believing they have little worth and do not deserve good things.
- As a terrified part of us that feels intensely afraid and unsafe – often a very young, non-verbal part that's felt intensely in the body.
- As a part that carries shame about who they are and what they choose.
- As a part that feels hopeless and despairing and that can see no way out.

In IFS these parts are called *exiles*, because they're the parts of us we push away. The ones I've given here are just examples – in reality, our exiles are unique to each of us. I've separated out the characteristics, but often we find that these characteristics belong to the same part. For example, the part that feels not enough may also be the part that carries shame about who they are.

Please pause for a moment before you continue reading and notice if this list has created activation in your system. I would expect it to – it's a lot to read, and it's likely that you will have identified with some of the parts I've described. Take some time to signal safety before you read on.

Protective parts are the voices, thoughts, beliefs and behaviours we experience the most. They're the top layer of parts. Their main purpose is to keep the wounded young parts that carry the trauma and pain out of conscious awareness. In the most counterintuitive of ways, protective parts aim to prevent us from feeling the intense emotion of our wounding. They are trying to safeguard us from things they perceive to be threatening. They work hard to control our relationships, our appearance, our attitude, our demeanour, our emotions, our behaviours and thoughts. They do this to avoid risk and ensure we don't get hurt. They fear what will happen if we're flooded by a wounded part and the trauma it carries. Protectors are child-like – they're young. It's important to remember that even ferocious, strong, adult-like protectors are still younger parts that are afraid and feeling threatened.

Examples of protective parts are: a judgemental part, an avoidant part, a 'need to figure it all out' part, a 'do more' perfectionist part, a compulsive eating part, a taskmaster part, a dismissive part, an endangerment part (which points out every possible danger and all the ways in which you're unsafe), a sceptical part, a people-pleasing part, a harsh bullying part, and a part that always asks, 'What's the point?'

If you're interested in your own protectors, take a moment to look back at your journalling work. See if you can spot your own protective ways of thinking and behaving. These adaptations and strategies *are* your protective parts.

Internal Family Systems (IFS) therapy uses a slightly more complicated model to explain traumatised parts. This model, although highly effective, can be a little too complex for self-led healing at home. Even differentiating two parts can at times feel unnecessary. As we undertake our own parts work at home, we aren't trying to categorise or figure out which part is which. Instead, and as you're going to learn and practise, we simply attend to whichever part is activated so we can anchor back into our adult self and help the part settle.

Parts work is glorious. It helps us experience our adult selves as separate from our wounded parts, allowing us to gain perspective and distance from our trauma and our wounding. It helps us more honestly meet ourselves and understand our inner world and psyche. It brings us into greater regulation, awareness, curiosity and compassion, and as it does, it helps us reinstate an anchoring adult into our inner world. As we learn to separate from our parts, we simultaneously gain space from our triggered reactions. Instead of reacting from a part, we become able to pause and choose how to respond from a place of self, and this is true empowerment and agency.

The Capacity Three Polarities
Here are the polarities that will help you get a better sense of what we're moving from and towards as we integrate Capacity Three:

- Part-led vs self-led
- Internalised abandonment vs internalised support
- Disconnected parts vs connected whole
- Triggered parts, in fear, vs soothed parts, in relationship
- Blended vs unblended[2]
- Child perspective vs adult perspective
- Reacting vs responding
- Criticism vs compassion
- Self-mistrust vs self-trust
- Resistance vs acceptance.

Take your time as you read through these polarities. Each one contains useful information about the journey we go on as we integrate Capacity Three. As we reinstate a compassionate, anchoring adult self, our experience of life changes, and self-trust deepens.

Self-led integration: A reminder

Continuing to integrate the other capacities is essential, not just to do parts work safely, but to do parts work at all. Separating from parts and anchoring back into self feels very hard if there's *only* dysregulation. As I explained previously (see Chapter Six), embodied safety allows us to integrate the other capacities. Capacity One is the foundation of this new way of being. As we increasingly move into the green zone, we experience a new sense of slowness and space internally. This slow spaciousness facilitates exploration of our inner world and our sense of self. Here, then, I'm reminding you of how essential increasing embodied safety is. Ensure you're continuing to signal safety as you do parts work by keeping aligned with principles Two, Five, Eight and Eleven:

- Principle One: Stretch don't stress – the 1 per cent rule.
- Principle Five: Find your way back to green.
- Principle Eight: Anchored connection heals us.
- Principle Eleven: Find soft places to land.

Moving into a parts approach is a big shift. It takes time to understand your inner world in this new way – you cannot gain perfect clarity about your parts and reinstate an anchoring adult quickly. Tomorrow, aim for 1 per cent more awareness and separation from your parts (Principle One). Gaining awareness of and being in relationship with your parts can feel *a lot*. Awareness of the younger parts of yourself that carry the trauma wounding can be particularly painful. For this reason, go slow (Principle One) and find your way back to green if/when the parts work feels too much (Principle Five). This can be achieved very simply by noticing that part of you is becoming distressed/activated by the parts work, pausing and signalling safety. Parts work helps us explore our inner worlds. If at any point your inner world feels too much for you, come out of the practice and anchor back into the real world using anchoring and connection tools (Principle Eight – see page 160).

The self-led approach I'm outlining here to create separation from parts and reinstate an anchoring adult works for many. But please get additional support from a trained IFS practitioner if you need it. This may be particularly necessary if you wish to do deeper healing work with wounded young parts. I've trained in IFS, but there are times that I need guidance in session from another IFS practitioner. I've heard many other exceptional IFS practitioners say the same. At times, we all need a trusted other to help us up the mountain and into resolution and release.

There are no prizes for struggling on alone (although I know your trauma makes you think there are). If you need help, guidance and support to integrate this capacity, get it (Principle Eleven).

Self

The concept of self comes alive in Capacity Three. Parts work allows us to see and separate from our traumatised parts (adaptations and wounding). As we unfold our parts, we naturally connect back to *self*. Self, then, exists underneath the wounding and the protective adaptations.

As we explore Capacity One, self is defined as the ventral vagal green zone. It's a regulated state we find our way back to. In Capacity Two, self is understood as a facet of conscious awareness – self as the seat of consciousness. Understanding self as we explore Capacity Three expands these previous definitions.

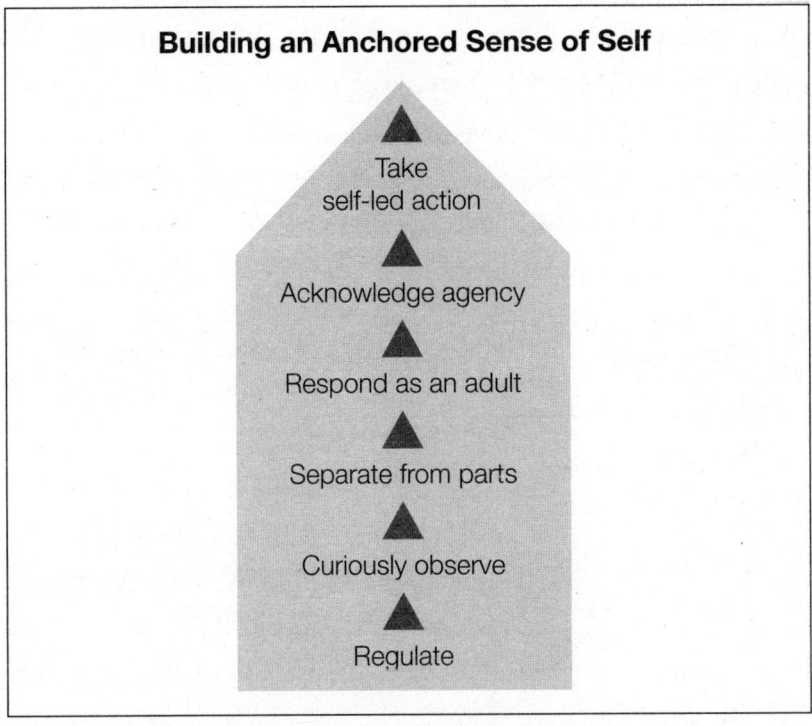

Diagram 5: Building an anchored sense of self

This diagram describes the process of building an anchored sense of self – starting from a foundation of greater regulation, we move into observation and curiosity and in turn can begin to separate from parts and respond to ourselves, our parts and our experiences from a place of adult perspective and compassion. As we anchor into our adult self, we become able to see and acknowledge our agency and increasingly take self-led action.

As we regulate and more easily move into curious observation, we become able to separate from our younger parts. As we then receive the younger parts of our psyche with perspective and compassion, we naturally reconnect to our adult self. *Adult* is the key term here. Parts are younger facets of our being that developed in the past. Our self is adult because it's us in the present moment – connected, curious and compassionate. Learning how to remain anchored into our adult self so we can become self-led rather than parts-led is trauma healing – it's the mountain top.

As well as describing how we understand self as we integrate Capacity Three, I'm also trying to give you a sense of how our experience of self develops and grows as we integrate the four capacities. Take a look at Diagram 5. The foundation of an anchored sense of self is signalling safety – it's found as we activate the ventral vagal nerve and regulate. As our nervous system moves out of patterns of dysregulation, survival and protection (such as anxiety or dissociation) we can more easily curiously observe ourselves and the world around us. As one of my clients said: 'Since doing the nervous system work it feels like there's a little more space and slowness internally, so I can see things more clearly.' As this space opens up to allow for greater curiosity and observation, we're then able to separate from our parts and operate from our adult self. Which in turn allow us to witness and integrate these parts into a cohesive sense of self. And as we anchor into our adult self, we move into agency and can increasingly take aligned, authentic action.

Internal Family Systems (IFS) refers to this magnificent, central part of our being simply as *self*. I interchangeably use the terms: self, adult self, core self, true self, wisest self and authentic self. Use whichever term feels true for you. Whatever you choose, you're describing *you* underneath the adaptations, dysregulation and trauma. The you that is:

- Connected
- Calm
- Present
- Curious
- Compassionate
- Equipped with adult perspective and reason
- Empowered.

Self, then, is the undamaged centre of us that exists underneath the parts. Strengthening our connection to self is central to healing our trauma. You're doing this already, of course. Every time you signal safety and regulate, you connect to self. Every time you separate from and curiously observe yourself, you connect to self. Parts work will strengthen this connection. Please note, the formal IFS concept of self is slightly broader, consisting of thirteen characteristics.

Before we move on I want to circle back to an idea I mentioned in Chapter Four – self as energy (see page 110). The concept of *self energy* is central to the IFS model, and it's a very helpful distinction for many as they begin to integrate Capacity Three. Self is a state (such as regulated, aware, open and present), but self is also an energy – a feeling that stems from, and can lead us back to, this *self state*. Reaching for just a little more *self energy* is a far gentler, kinder, more realistic aim than trying to move from chronic dysregulation straight into a regulated *self state*. Try to remember that self exists as an energy you can reach for at any moment of the day. These characteristics of self are your guide to pulling some of this *self energy* into a moment:

- Connection to your body, the world and others brings in self energy.
- Calm brings in self energy.
- Presence brings in self energy.
- Curiosity brings in self energy.
- Compassion brings in self energy.
- A reasonable adult perspective brings in self energy.
- Acknowledging your agency brings in self energy.

No matter what you're doing or where you are, you can anchor back into self by pulling in more self energy. As you do, you'll move out of autopilot and protective patterns and into awareness and expansion.

Experiencing self

For the next 24 hours play around with the concept of self. Self is a regulated state of connection and presence *and* it's an energy/feeling. Self emerges as you relate to, see and separate from your experiences and parts. It's you underneath the reactive, protective parts. As you move into connection, calm, presence, curiosity, compassion, perspective and agency, you separate from your parts and move into self energy.

Being in self feels expansive and open, light and relaxed – this is because self is also the ventral vagal green zone. Although we're using the language of self, you're utilising a lot of capacities you've already started to integrate – signalling safety, presence, observation and curiosity.

Play with these ideas to help you get an experiential sense of self. Try to notice when you're in self, even if it's just for a fleeting moment. Over time aim to build an experiential, embodied sense of how it feels to be in self. Also try to get a sense of self-led actions you can take to increase self-energy – remember that practising any of the facets of self (connection, calm, presence, etc.) will do this.

Clusters of parts

There are many different *parts* models. The addiction specialist and author Pia Mellody's adaptive child model and Schwartz's Internal Family Systems (IFS) model are two of the leading ones people working with childhood trauma often use. Both are powerful descriptors of our inner world and guides to healing. The beauty of the IFS model is that it encourages us to see how our parts operate together – as an *internal family system*. The model encourages us to curiously observe our inner world, our reactions, thoughts, behaviours, emotions and beliefs so we can get an overarching sense of the entire *system* of parts. Where other parts models tell us precisely which parts are in there (an inner child, an inner critic, an adaptive child and so on), the IFS model gives us creative freedom. We're encouraged to describe our inner world of parts as it is, rather than trying to squeeze our internal experience into a set format. This leads to greater authenticity and self-acceptance.

In *No Bad Parts*, Schwartz explains that people have a vast number of parts that are separate from the Self. This proliferation of parts is completely normal. Coming to see and accept them is a main goal of what we're trying to do here. We aim to see and move into relationships with the individual parts, but also to understand how parts are operating together.

In any given situation, or underneath any triggered reaction, we'll find clusters of parts. The people-pleasing part example I mentioned above illustrates this. The triggered people-pleasing (fawn) part was the part that caught our attention, but as we looked closer, we found another part that was exhausted and had had enough of people-pleasing. There was also a younger part that was afraid they were 'unlovable'. The protectors were triggered alongside the young, wounded part to try to keep it safe.

Parts never operate in isolation. There are always multiple parts that hold different, often opposing, positions. This is particularly true when you're experiencing extreme tension, overwhelm or inner conflict. If you become aware of a part that, say, wants to give up, when you look closer you may find another part that urges you to keep going and do more. The opposing parts are creating the inner tension and conflict. Often these polarised parts are the root cause of freeze and paralysis. One of the main reasons IFS has become a leading treatment model for childhood trauma is that the concepts of multiple parts and polarised parts are intuitively easy to understand and apply.

Before you move into observation of your parts, be mindful that there are always multiple parts. Seeing and separating from the clusters of parts brings clarity and relief.

Step One: Separating and unblending

As part of the new self-led way of being you're developing, we aim to separate and *unblend* from our younger, wounded and protective parts. We do this so we can experience a sense of separation from our trauma and bring some healing (through relationship) to our parts. We also do this so we can live life in a self-led rather than parts-led way. For many, this idea can feel confusing and even triggering, because a lot of us totally identify with our parts. We can't separate our self from our inner child, say. There's no space: we're merged and entwined with all the familiar, reactive, hurt parts of ourselves. If the cruel, unkind, self-hating voice of your critical part is so familiar that it feels like it IS your voice, it's going to take time to separate from it, and that's okay. This will click. There will be a moment where you feel a glorious sense of relief as you experience a sense of separation from your parts, even those that currently feel so familiar you think of them as 'who you really are'.

Initially, separating and unblending is about noticing activation and then moving into the language of *parts*. Remember that anything that is not self (connected, calm, present, curious, compassionate, 'adult', empowered) is a part. When you notice a familiar way of thinking, state of mind, behaviour or emotion has been activated, once again pause and move into curious observation, but this time refer to the experience as a 'part'. This could sound like:

- 'Part of me is feeling so sad today – I wonder why.'
- 'Part of me urgently wants to figure everything out – isn't that interesting.'
- 'The part of me that wants to eat and eat and eat is very strong today – I wonder why this part is so activated.'
- 'I feel deeply anxious today – I wonder if I'm blended with a part that feels unsafe.'
- 'Part of me feels so so sad today.'

- 'Part of me feels like a failure today – it's such a strong feeling, I wonder why.'

Subtly changing your language and making these observations in a curious and compassionate way brings more *self energy* to the moment.

Step Two: Getting a sense of the part

Once we've created just a little air gap between our adult self and the younger part, we next try to get a better sense of the part. This helps us continue to separate and anchor back into self. Sometimes as we do this work we see an image of a part; sometimes it's a feeling in our body or a sense that the part is 'here'. In IFS, they refer to this stage as fleshing out the part. For example, describing the part that feels like a failure could sound like:

- I can feel the part in my chest – it's so tight.
- The part feels like they're getting everything wrong – I can feel it in the pit of my stomach and as racing anxiety in my chest.
- The part feels so much shame – I can feel it in my body.
- This part is so afraid.
- This part is showing me images of times in the past when I got things wrong.
- I can see an image of this part – she's young and curled up in a ball trying to hide.

If it feels more natural, you can directly acknowledge the part by addressing it as 'you' whenever you get a sense of it, as I describe in the next section – something like 'I can feel *your* fear in my chest.' There's no right or wrong here, and as you move into self-led parts work at home, you'll find what feels natural for you. All that matters here is that you pause to connect with what the part is feeling and experiencing. Use whatever language feels right for you.

Step Three: Into relationship

There are many ways we can take self-led action to heal our younger parts. To guide this work, we remember that parts become extreme because they are out of connection (feeling alone and unanchored) and sensing threat (feeling unsafe). Healing, then, is all about bringing parts back into connection and relationship and helping them feel safer.

One of the gentlest, most beautiful ways to do this, creating settling in our system and bringing some healing self energy to our parts, is to give them what has been missing – acknowledgement, understanding and validation. Taking self-led action to see, hear, understand and validate a part that's been activated is deeply healing. As another subtle shift of language, we address the part directly, using 'you'. This could sound like:

- 'I can see you now.'
- 'I see you feel like you've made a mistake.'
- 'I see you, I'm here.'
- 'I know you feel afraid.'
- 'I know it's hard right now.'
- 'I understand why you feel this way.'
- 'It makes sense that you feel this way.'

Step Four: Reassuring parts

If it feels comfortable to do so, providing the part with connection and reassurance will also help it settle. This could sound like:

- 'I'm not going anywhere, it's okay.'
- 'I know you feel afraid, it's okay, I'm here, everything's going to be okay.'
- 'I know you feel you need to protect me, but we're safe, there's no emergency.'
- 'I'm listening now, you're not alone.'

We integrate Capacity Three by practising separating from and then responding to our parts with this new, compassion-ate adult response. Over time, the response I'm describing (separating, seeing, hearing, acknowledging, validating and reassuring parts) can reinstate self as the anchoring adult in your inner system. Gently and respectfully, we give our younger parts what they need by validating their experiences and reassuring them (as a loving parent would).

As we integrate Capacity Three, our inner system of parts moves into conscious awareness and clarity. And we (as self) become captain of the ship – able to separate from and soothe reactive parts so we can live life from self.

Step Five: Regulating with parts

Once you've created some separation from the part and then acknowledged and validated its feelings and experience, move into one of your soothing techniques, but do this *with* the part. This could look like:

- Asking the part to breathe with you.
- Visualising the part sitting next to you and asking it to hear the sound of you 'voooooooo-ing'.

For more of these soothing techniques, see page 185. Any of these techniques can be done with an activated part to create connection and help the part settle. This might sound weird, I know. But the joy of parts work is that it can sound strange until we experience it – then it feels like we've hit upon the secret to mental health and healing.

The corrective experience

As I've described the five steps, I've given lots of wording to describe the process we move through as we do healing parts work at home:

- Step One: Unblending
- Step Two: Getting a sense of the part
- Step Three: Seeing and validating the part
- Step Four: Reassuring the part
- Step Five: Regulating/soothing with the part

In reality, it's not so structured and scripted. This is one of the hardest things about the self-led approach: it's about experien tial learning. We learn as we take action. As you start practising these ideas and principles, you'll get a feel for it and make it your own.

As a guide to this process, I just want to remind you that you're trying to give your younger parts (the protective adap-tations and the wounded child parts) a *corrective* experience.

What this means is that you're giving them a contrasting experience to what they received in childhood. So, if as a child you (and therefore your parts) were met with criticism rather than compassion, you give them a corrective experience by showing them only compassion. This idea of giving a corrective experience leads to deep healing because we're being called to move out of our autopilot and trauma-led patterns. It's hard because we have to do the opposite of how we've been conditioned. But because we're doing that, it heals us and move us out of trauma patterns. This, by the way, is the primary function of most psychotherapeutic approaches – the therapist aims to give you a corrective experience, such as an opportunity to express difficult feelings and have them heard, and in doing so help you heal. The IFS and self-led way help you give yourself this experience.

Take some time now to think about how you (and your parts) were received as children. This gives you important information on how to give yourself a corrective experience.

Examples of childhood experience vs corrective experience

Childhood	Corrective
Rushed	Slow
Absence	Presence
Ignored	Seen
Cruelty	Kindness
Dismissed	Acknowledged
Impatience	Patience
Rejected	Accepted
Criticism	Praise
Unloved	Loved
Tough	Gentle

Use this table to get a sense of what you need to give your parts to help them have a corrective experience, and therefore move into healing. In practice, this is the hard edge of healing. If, say, you're conditioned to ignore vulnerability, you will need to very slowly build your capacity to see, be with and accept your parts' vulnerability. Take your time, and remember to dip in and out of the discomfort (Principle Four).

Parts interrupting parts work

As you try to get a sense of a part, try to notice if other parts of you pop up. This is likely, as parts of us tend to be grouped into clusters – multiple parts are triggered by similar situations, or when one part activates, its distress/energy activates another part. To do this, try to notice any resistance, emotions, thoughts or sensations that are triggered by you trying to separate/explore a part.

This could sound like:

- I feel afraid – I think the part of me that feels afraid has been activated by doing this IFS work.
- I can feel myself getting very frustrated at the part of me that feels like a failure. I wonder if that's a different part – I think a frustrated part has been activated.
- I'm starting to dissociate and feel dizzy – I think a checking-out part has been activated because it feels too much.

IFS teaches us that a tip for checking if a part is interrupting parts work is to pause and ask yourself: 'How do I feel towards this part?' For example, if you're connecting with the part of you that's a compulsive doer, pause and ask yourself: 'How do I feel towards this compulsive doer part?' If you feel compassionate, curious, calm or neutral towards the part then you're in self energy. If you feel anything else (angry, afraid, disgusted) then it means another part of you has been triggered by the work. The feeling (and the thoughts that accompany the feeling) *is* the part that's interrupted parts work. Acknowledge this new part of you that's popped up. This could sound like:

- 'I can see you – it's okay, I understand why you're afraid of the compulsive doer part. I get it.'
- 'I can feel you – I understand why you feel angry towards the compulsive doer part.'

Next, ask this new part of you to separate a little so you can continue communicating with the 'target' part. You can literally speak directly to the new part that's been activated – see, hear, acknowledge and validate it – and ask the part if they're willing to unblend a little so you can continue with your work. This could sound like:

- 'I know you're angry, but could you unblend just a little so I can carry on talking with the compulsive doer part?'
- 'I understand why you're here. Could you come and sit next to me so I can carry on with this work?'

If they won't, that's okay too – continue to validate and reassure the new part. Make this new part that popped up the part you're giving attention to, but also take a moment to communicate what you're doing with the original part – this could sound like, 'I need to spend some time with this part, but I want to connect with you too – I'm on my way to you.'

Separating and unblending from the cluster of parts brings in self energy and helps us regulate. Always remember the lead principle here: find your way back to the green zone. Use any tools (soothing, anchoring and connection techniques) as well as the characteristics of self (curiosity and compassion) to bring you towards the green zone during self-led parts work if it feels too much.

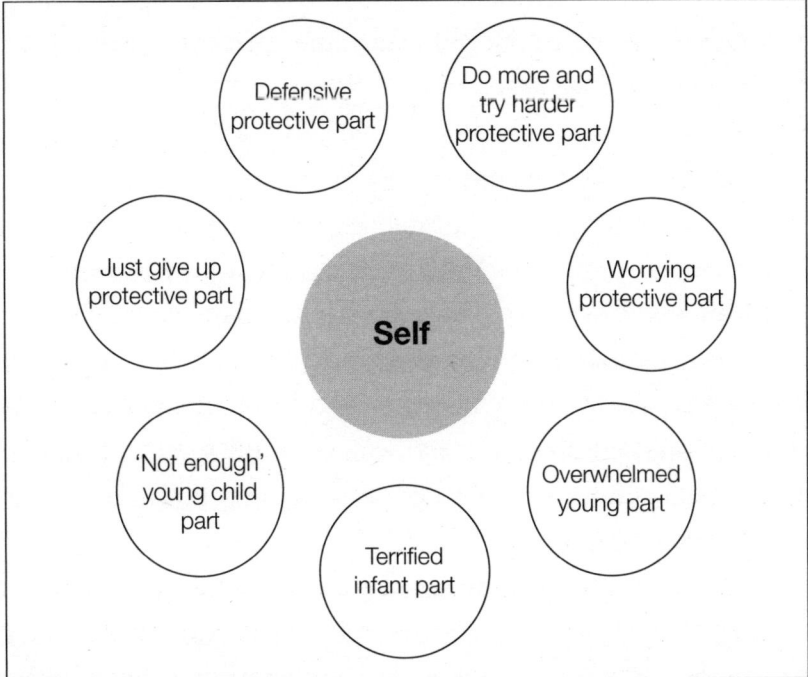

Diagram 6: Parts mapping

Illustrates the multiple wounded and protective parts of a client's inner world that were triggered because of conflict at work. Mapping our parts in this way helps us see the conflict between the different parts of us – with one part here calling them to give up, and another part calling them to do more and try harder.

Parts mapping

A nice way into this work is to start mapping your parts. I've included Diagram 6 to show you how one of my clients did this. Rob mapped out his parts on a piece of scrap paper a few days before our session. He'd done this to get some perspective and clarity because he was experiencing overwhelm and felt flooded by a conflict at work. He mapped three wounded young parts and four protective parts. The young parts of Rob that believe they're not enough and feel intensely terrified were triggered by the work conflict. The protective parts of him took over to try and push down the painful thoughts, feelings and beliefs that belong to the old wounding. When he showed me this he said:

> It feels very odd seeing myself on paper like that – this little scrap of paper accurately describes my daily inner experience. It's what it's like to be me, and why it's so hard to get anything done. There are parts in there pulling me in so many different directions.

Parts mapping is a self-led action we can do daily to bring us into greater conscious awareness and reconnect us to our adult self. It's particularly helpful when we're really in it, flooded by old adaptations and wounding. If you feel like the walls are closing in, grab a piece of paper and write down all the parts of you that are activated. The effect can be instant – bringing a sense of clarity, adult perspective and regulation.

Existential crisis

At one point or another all my clients look at me with fear in their eyes and ask: 'But who am I if I'm no longer all these adaptations and parts?' As terrifying as this thought is, I know they're near the top of the mountain when they experientially move into this realisation. Initially, we experience relief from separating and unblending; then it becomes something of an existential crisis.

Parts are familiar. They give us our sense of identity and provide our rulebook for relating to the world. Yes, we all want to stop operating from a people-pleasing part, say, or an anxious part. But then what? What exists in place of these familiar, automatic ways of being? Well, *self* is what exists underneath these things.

Self is glorious – it is a place of calm, curiosity, presence and compassion. Being in your adult self (present, connected, aware and curious) means you can increasingly connect to your own authentic truths – your limits, wants, needs and values. From this new anchored authenticity you can start creating life rather than reacting to it. Being in self gives us a radically different experience of life and relationships. But this difference is unsettling. In many ways self is unsettling – without the highs and lows, without the extremeness of parts, this new calm state of presence and connection feels very odd indeed.

So odd, in fact, that this new absence of internal reactions can feel very much as if there's a problem. A story from my own healing journey illustrates this beautifully.

During a therapy session with my own IFS therapist, I cried as I said I was certain that I had early onset dementia. My lovely, extremely patient therapist asked me to describe and explain why part of me held this fear. I went on to describe how different conversations now felt. 'Before I was on the edge of my seat – I knew where the conversation was heading and I'd jump in with an answer or a joke before the person had even finished their sentence. I was so quick and so certain.

'But now I just sit there. I'm not preparing an answer – sometimes I don't even have anything to say.'

I sobbed and my therapist nodded in that sage way that therapists do. After some time she gently said:

'So, am I right that now you're actually listening to the other person, instead of half listening, while full of adrenaline and composing a perfect answer?'

'Yes,' I said as I felt that unnerving 'my therapist's on to something' feeling.

She continued: 'You're listening. Okay. And do you feel calm and present as the other person is talking?'

'Yes,' I said.

'And then you take a moment before you respond?' she asked.

'Yes,' I said again.

'And sometimes you have nothing to say, you're just receiving the information?'

'Yes,' I said one last time, feeling as if a trick was being played on me.

Finally my therapist said: 'This sounds very much like you're regulated and in self during conversations now. This does not, to me, sound like early onset dementia. But it sounds as if part, or parts of you, are deeply afraid of this change.'

I cannot explain the joy and lightness I felt as my therapist pointed out the blindingly obvious. As soon as she mirrored back to me my experience, I heard the truth – that I was in self, and that far from illness there was healing, but part of me was deeply afraid of this new way of connecting.

This interaction highlights two things. Firstly, it reveals that moving into regulation, awareness and self-connection is a weird, unnerving journey at times. This is particularly true within relationships where *doing it differently* can at times feel uncomfortable and at other times feel deeply unsafe. Secondly, it beautifully demonstrates that at times we cannot see the wood for the trees (the self for the parts) so we need someone else to see and hear our parts, and hold the adult perspective for us.

Deeper healing practices

To help you get a better sense of separation from your parts, and to help these parts heal through resolution and release, we can use deeper healing practices.

I find this deeper healing work is most effective as an occasional practice rather than woven into the day-to-day. But as you gain in confidence, you may feel able to pull some of these approaches into daily life.

These practices are safe, providing you're applying the Principles of Self-led Integration and, of course, that they don't feel too much for you. If they do cross your line of 'too much', find a trained IFS practitioner to work with.

Practice One: Good morning

This gentle morning practice is lovely. I use it often. To start with, take a couple of minutes to regulate and signal safety to your nervous system. Once you feel a sense of settling, start this parts exercise. I do this cross-legged as I would a meditation, but sitting or lying down works just as well.

Put your hand on your heart, and if it feels safe to, close your eyes. Move into curious observation and the parts approach by asking yourself: 'Good morning, who needs my attention today? I'm here and I'm listening.'

You may find you immediately notice a familiar part of you. If not, curiously observe your body and mind, and name the parts that are present slowly and consciously, welcoming each part to the new day. This could sound like:

'Hi, I see you.'

If you sense that a part is in need of a longer, deeper connection or is in a lot of distress, focus on this part (see, hear, acknowledge, validate, reassure).

Before you come out of the practice, see if you can hold all the parts you've welcomed in mind and send healing love and light to them, by visualising flowing, loving light from your heart to them. When you're ready to come out of the practice, thank the parts for showing up and say goodbye.

Practice Two: Into the safe space

This is an extension of the safe space visualisation I describe in Appendix B. For a reminder, head there now to begin to use your own imagination to develop your own safe space. For this practice, you're going to invite your parts into your safe space with you, as Naomi did with her mother garden.

As above, to begin, take a couple of minutes to regulate and signal safety to your nervous system. Once you feel it begin to settle, start this exercise. Again, I do this sitting cross-legged on the floor, but sitting or lying however you feel comfortable is fine.

Put your hand on your heart, and if it feels safe to, close your eyes. Bring to mind your safe space. Take your time doing this. Once you feel the sense of regulation this space brings, invite in a part that you want to soothe and get to know. If the part doesn't want to, or you struggle to do this, don't worry. In this instance, talk to the part – ask it to see you there and tell it it's welcome to join you in this safe lovely nourishing space whenever it wants to.

If you do sense or see that the part is now in the safe space with you, let it put itself anywhere it wants to be. Don't tell it what to do. Communicate with an energy of loving respect and curiosity. Once the part is in the space, communicate with it (see, hear, acknowledge, validate, reassure) and send love and compassion to it. If it doesn't want to receive the care and compassion, that's okay. Just be with this part in this space. If it feels comfortable to, you can communicate with this part – asking it what it needs from you or what it's afraid of. When you're ready to come out of the space, thank the part for showing up and being with you before you say goodbye to it.

Remember as you do this to check if other parts have been activated by asking yourself: 'How do I feel towards this part?' If you realise another part has been activated by the parts work, take a moment to unblend from the part.

Practice Three: Getting to know a protective part

This practice is an extension of the five-step process I outlined on page 251. Use this if you want to get to know a protective part better after you've unblended, got a sense of the part and validated it. Remember to check if any other parts are present before you begin. Try asking the part some of the following questions:

- 'What are you trying to protect me from?'
- 'When did you first start doing this for me?'
- 'What made you take on this role?'
- 'What are you afraid would happen if you stopped doing this job?'
- 'How do you feel?'
- 'What do you need?'

Listen with curiosity and compassion, acknowledge and validate the protective part's efforts, and thank them for so tirelessly trying to keep you safe.

Practice Four: Healing a wounded part

The wounded young parts of us feel different to the protective parts of us. They're vulnerable and in pain. Some clients are almost solely living within protective parts; others are almost completely blended with wounded young parts. Others oscillate between the two. This practice is designed to bring healing self energy to wounded parts – the very young, little parts of you that are feeling intense emotions and holding damaging beliefs.

This healing practice is not something to rush towards. Do this after you've been practising parts work for a while, and only once you've got a good sense of your protective parts and how it feels to be in your adult self. And you may find it safest to do with a practitioner, so you can feel supported by the therapist's regulated adult self.

First, try to get a sense of the wounded part. You may feel the part as an emotion or sensation in your body (such as fear, panic, terror, shame, anger or sadness), or you may get a sense of them or a visual image or hear them in your mind. Invite the young wounded part to sit next to you or to place themselves anywhere they want to be. Some find it very helpful to visualise their safe space and invite the wounded part into the space. Sometimes young parts are scared to be seen. Don't force them to show themselves – allow them to be hidden if they feel safest this way. Thank the part for being clear with you and reassure them that it's okay.

It's likely that this connection with the deeper wounded parts of yourself will trigger other parts. Protective parts wary of you getting too close to your emotional pain could become activated or other wounded parts may show up. You might start trying to 'figure it out' intellectually, or feel anxious, afraid, irritated or so on. If you notice something else is present, pause the work. Mentally turn towards the part that's been activated.

Never bypass, ignore or push through protective parts of yourself – always acknowledge them and ask permission to continue with the deeper work. If your protectors are hesitant or say no, try and understand why. Address the fears or hesitancy by acknowledging them, then reassure the protector that you're here to help them and the wounded part. If it's a strong 'no' from a protective part of you, listen to it and thank it for doing its job so well. Before you move out of parts work, gently communicate with the young wounded part that you'll be back soon. If it feels right to, visualise putting the young vulnerable part somewhere safe and nourishing. Say goodbye to both the protective part and the wounded part before you leave the practice.

If you sense that the protective part of you has softened and is willing for you to continue connecting to the wounded young part of yourself, thank it and ask it to continue to unblend and stand next to you or move to the side.

Next, connect to the young, vulnerable part. See, validate and reassure, as outlined in the steps above on pages 246 to 251. If the young part is responding and open to communicating with you, ask them if they want to tell or show you anything. You may see an image of something or hear words. No matter what the images or words are, validate, reassure and thank the part for showing you this and trusting you. If a confused part or 'figure it out' part pops up, notice and unblend. Use self-regulation techniques to hold yourself through and remain connected to self if need be. Also remember that moving into curiosity or compassion will naturally connect you back to your adult self – so bringing more of this energy will help you stay present and connected. This is important. Take time to signal safety to ensure you can hold yourself, and the wounded part, through any discomfort.

If at any point this work feels too much, tell the wounded part that you need to slow things down to keep them, and yourself, safe. Ask the wounded part to unblend a little. Literally, ask them not to flood you – explain you can help them more if they unblend just a little. It can be helpful to visualise them outside of yourself, somewhere in the safe space or sitting next to you. If you're able to move yourself and your wounded part towards the green zone, carry on with the practice. If not (if you feel flooded), say goodbye to the child part and come out of this inner parts work. Use the safety-signalling tools to help yourself regulate. If this doesn't ease things, take this as a sign that you need co-regulation (a regulated adult to help your system move back into safety).

Once you have witnessed some of the wounded part's emotions or beliefs, ask the part what it needs and how you can help it. Listen and acknowledge any requests that it makes. Finally, visualise putting this part somewhere they'll feel safe. Do this with an energy of compassion and love. They may want to stay in the safe space, they may want to be wrapped in a protective bubble of golden light. They may need a cuddle, or they may want to go somewhere safe and snuggly (like a little den). Give them whatever you sense will help them feel safe as you move out of the practice.

When you're ready to come out of the work, thank the part for showing up and being with you before you say goodbye to it. Check in with this wounded part during the next 48 hours – drop in to connection with it and remind it that you see it now and it's not alone any more.

Self-led trauma healing

Another practitioner working in this field and fascinated by the idea of self-healing is Dr Jay Earley. Jay is a psychologist and a huge proponent of using IFS at home to self-heal. His work is bold and interesting. Jay, like me, is highlighting that there's much we can do to heal our own trauma. In *Self-Therapy*, Jay writes: 'Whenever you endure a painful or difficult experience, it must be fully processed and metabolised for your psyche to stay healthy.'[3] To heal, he believes you must 'feel the experience, make sense of it, integrate it into your notion of who you are in a way that doesn't leave you with a negative, inaccurate view of yourself.'

Here, Jay is explaining how we heal our parts and our trauma – by witnessing their pain and experience from an adult perspective and allowing their feelings to be present alongside compassion and adult care. Our adult self makes sense of (processes and understands) the childhood experience. Our adult self also allows some of the feelings to move through us, alongside compassion and in a way that feels safe, by signalling safety, pendulating, unblending, and pulling in the self energy of curiosity and compassion.

Traditionally, this is the role of the therapist: they witness and provide a corrective experience. The therapist also endeavours to help us feel some of our pain in a safe way – moving us gently from contraction to release and resolution. In many ways then, this concept of the adult self as the witness, a corrective relationship, and as safely guiding the emotional experience puts us in the position of being our own therapist and healer.

This book is about the revolution that's unfolding – about how multiple modalities are handing the power of healing back to each of us. IFS, along with Somatic Experiencing (SE) and the polyvagal approach, are all powerful trauma healing modalities. Working with practitioners who have trained in them is, in my experience, a new, expansive kind of therapeutic experience. This is because these modalities are inherently empowering. They recognise the power of self-led action and aim to teach us how to stand in, own and connect to our power to self-heal through internal and external action.

The capacities in this book are designed to help you connect to your adult self, so you too can create real change and deep healing for yourself. As Richard Schwartz so aptly stated in the title of his most recent book: *you* are the one you've been waiting for.[4]

Working with a practitioner

Although the IFS parts approach can be used as a tool for self-healing, many benefit from working with a practitioner. The self-led approach is not a masochistic exercise in hyper-independence, endurance and pushing through. In fact, moving into these adaptations indicates that you're no longer stretching and shaping, and instead are stressed (Principle One) – something feels too much and is moving you into survival.

I recommend that you work with an IFS-trained practitioner if you:

- Are struggling to integrate Capacity One – for example, if over time you feel there's no increase in your capacity to regulate or your connection to your body
- Have parts that are engaged in extreme behaviours
- Have parts that are in extreme emotional distress
- Feel that you need support to safely explore your inner world
- Struggle to separate and unblend from parts
- Sense that there are buried/inaccessible parts
- Want to do more to heal wounded parts.

Choosing to work with a practitioner doesn't take away your power to self-heal – it facilitates it. Please also remember, as Sheryl Close highlighted in Chapter Five, that you may benefit from working with a somatic trauma practitioner to create more co-regulation in your system before you engage in IFS work.

Chapter Nine

Capacity four: unlocking your agency and taking self-led action

You've already been taking action, so a chapter designed to help you take action may seem a little . . . unnecessary. But this capacity is about increasingly taking real-world action, rather than the internal action we take to help move us into the green zone, curiously observe, separate from our wounded parts and connect to self. Here, then, we're thinking about how to take authentic, aligned self-led action in the world around us. We're moving from self-led action that aims to effect change internally to self-led action that aims to effect change externally.

This capacity is built on the previous ones. We become able to connect to our agency and take self-led action in the world around us as we increasingly regulate, move into curious observation and separate from the younger parts of our psyche so we can anchor into our adult self. As we take self-led action to integrate Capacities One, Two and Three, connecting to and operating from *self* becomes increasingly possible. First, self emerges and then it becomes our home base. This home base becomes our anchor and our guide, giving us direction and intention as we take action in life.

Self-led action is spontaneous, free, responsive and anchored into the ventral vagal *self state*. It feels aligned with our adult limits, wants, needs and values. This type of action stands in direct contrast to trauma-led action, which we take when we're triggered and operating from a wounded or protective part/adaptation. Self-led action is a *response* that we can choose because we're regulated, aware and in our adult self. Trauma-led action is a *reaction* driven by subconscious autopilot, dysregulation and our younger parts.

Self-led action is powered by our sense of agency – an embodied feeling of freedom, empowerment and choice. Action is the outcome; agency is the gentle power that drives it. Agency is often wrongly conflated with control, but they're not quite the same thing. Aiming to feel or be 'in control' can be problematic for those with childhood trauma. Making it our goal can lead us into old fear-led patterns that don't serve us. A need for control can quickly move from an expansive, 'I've got this' energy into a rigid, fixed survival energy that pulls us further into dysregulation as we inevitably veer between feeling unsafe and out of control to becoming overly protective and controlling. Whereas aiming to feel and acknowledge our agency moves us into patterns of connection and expansion, leading to greater regulation and an increased sense of safety.

Agency is an embodied feeling of freedom, empowerment and choice. These feelings become more and more available to us as we make our way towards the mountain top. Agency emerges as we build an anchored sense of self. As we signal safety, regulate, move into greater awareness and separate from our parts, we interrupt subconscious trauma-led patterns.

We move from autopilot, with limited choice about how we behave, feel, relate and experience life, into agency – an anchored sense that we have the freedom to choose. Trauma disconnects us from our agency because it locks us into patterns and takes away our choice. Trauma healing reconnects us to our agency as we step out of these patterns and become able to choose. Self-led trauma healing is particularly well placed to increase agency because it calls you to choose and implement actions every single day. As you do, your sense of agency slowly re-establishes.

If you've already started practising this approach, you may have experienced a greater sense of agency and choice. Perhaps you've noticed it during a moment of regulation that allowed you to pause rather than rush in. Or perhaps it happened as you separated from your younger parts, anchored back into adult you, and were able to respond in a new way. This feeling of space and choice is agency.

Agency matters in the world of trauma healing because it moves us out of autopilot. But it also matters because it increases our sense of self-efficacy – our belief in ourselves and our capacity to create change. Self-efficacy is knowing we can do something. It's self-belief.

Agency (I can choose) and self-efficacy (I can do this) feed into each other – they're two sides of the same coin. Experiencing and deepening both is essential for childhood trauma healing, because the wounding and protective adaptations of childhood trauma erode both.

Integrating Capacity Four is about moving into agency and increasing self-efficacy in a more conscious way – acknowledging and increasing this expansive feeling. It's also about using your agency to take self-led action that moves you consciously in the direction you want to go. A direction that's authentically aligned with who you truly are: with self.

The Capacity Four Polarities

This whole book is designed to help you differentiate between your true self and your trauma, because until we begin to do this, we're lost in the fog of autopilot and trauma-led patterns. These polarities help you differentiate so you can get a sense of where your self begins and ends, and where your trauma begins and ends. Here are the polarities that will help you get a better sense of what you're moving from and to as you integrate Capacity Four:

- Trauma-led action vs self-led action
- Disempowered vs empowered
- Autopilot vs agency
- Adaptations vs authenticity
- Misaligned with limits, wants, needs and values vs aligned with limits, wants, needs and values
- Reacting vs creating
- No choice vs choice.

Self-led integration: A reminder

As you integrate Capacity Four and move into agency and action, it's so very important that you keep practising the Principles of Self-led Integration. As you increasingly take action in the world, it's important to remain anchored into self and into the new way of being you're creating.

The principles that are particularly relevant as you integrate Capacity Four are principles One, Two, Five, Nine and Ten:

- Principle One: Stretch don't stress.
- Principle Two: Experiment and play to find what works.
- Principle Five: Find your way back to green.
- Principle Nine: Acknowledge your agency.
- Principle Ten: Allow your inner wisdom to guide you.

As you move into action, find your growth edge – that beautiful line that indicates that you're stretching and growing. But don't do too much too soon – slow is fast in trauma healing (Principle One). More so than in any of the other capacities, here in Capacity Four it's essential that you give yourself permission to experiment and play to find flow, what you like, what you need, what you value and what you want to create (Principle Two). As always, continue to make the green zone home base to ensure you keep moving back into release and expansion (Principle Five). Capacity Four is all about agency and empowerment. This idea is encapsulated in Principle Nine – so use it often as you begin to take self-led action in life. Finally, and beautifully, as you make changes and take action, remain in connection with self so you can be guided by your own wisdom (Principle Ten).

Control vs serenity

Trauma responses are incomplete nervous system survival processes that result from feeling threatened. But they also occur because we sense that the threat is too much for us to handle. In other words, the traumatic reaction is a response to feeling, and often being, out of control. Because of this, all protective adaptations are designed to help us feel in control in some way. Think about people-pleasing, rumination, tension

and contraction in the body, undereating, overeating, avoidance, minimising, self-blame or perfectionism – they all help
us cope by giving us back some semblance of control. In
reality we are not in control. We are reacting, manipulating
and clinging on tight to avoid reality.

Our trauma and protective adaptations have decided that
being in *control* is the ultimate goal. It's what we're all attempting to attain, day in, day out. More control, by any means
necessary, to counteract the vulnerable wounding at our
centre. From our trauma's point of view, complete control is
the mountain top – the vision of security it has decided we
need to be safe.

Only it's impossible. It's a mountain top we'll never reach,
because it doesn't exist – so much of life is out of our control.
I don't enjoy writing this. I want to claim the opposite – to tell
you that you can manifest extreme powers of control if you
just try harder. But I also know that your healing relies on
you becoming able to tolerate the uncomfortable truth I've just
outlined.

The sense of control our protective adaptations give us is
fake. It soothes us or gives us a sense of power and domination, but it's not actually control. It's a fear-based reaction. So
what's the solution? What do we reach for once we accept this?
The answer is agency, because although complete control is
never available to us, agency is always and endlessly *ours*.

In the midst of a triggered reaction, a challenging moment
at work, a crisis, a conflict, a hard day, we need to acknowledge
and unlock our agency. We achieve this by signalling safety,
getting curious, and receiving ourselves with perspective and
compassion because these new ways of living interrupt the
protective reactions that are desperately seeking control. But we

also achieve it when we consider what we can realistically change – what we need to accept and let go of, and where we can effect change.

The serenity prayer is the cornerstone of the 12-step approach: 'Grant me the serenity to accept the things I cannot change, the courage to change the things I can, and the wisdom to know the difference.'

For a time, this short prayer was my entire daily program. Every day, for months, it guided me away from trauma-led action and into self-led action that would help me heal and grow. Perhaps this time spent teaching myself to acknowledge what I can and cannot change is why I now passionately believe that it's essential for trauma healing. Why I can see that acknowledging our agency is fundamental to trauma healing and real change.

Even today, as I repeat this prayer to myself, life suddenly becomes very clear indeed. I see where I'm clinging on, but need to let go. I also see what I can choose to change. As I say the words of this prayer today, my inner wisdom shows me what I need to know: I cannot change the past. I cannot change what I said on Saturday. I cannot change the choices I made twenty years ago. I cannot change the choice I made six years ago. I cannot change the economy. I cannot change the people in my life.

I *can* change how I speak to myself. I can change my attitude. I can choose to respond from my adult self. I can choose to trust myself. I can choose to stay on my own side. I can change how much I self-care today.

This breakdown of my life into things I can and cannot change is highly reassuring. As I note to myself what lies outside of my control, something in me settles. The protective parts and adaptations that were clinging on let go just a little.

This list, written by my adult self, provides these parts with an adult perspective that soothes them.

As you heal, you get to choose how you show up. You get to make a choice about the words that come out of your mouth. You get to choose how you relate to a person and a problem. You get to choose whether you self-care. You have a choice about whether you stay or go, whether you act or don't act. Your response and your relationship to a situation, person or problem is the only part of the life-equation that you can truly *control*.

The serenity prayer is far more than a prayer. It's a way of moving into self-led, aligned, adult action and away from trauma-led autopilot, wounding and adaptations. This alone, without all the guidance and practices I'm including in this chapter, will help you move into agency and self-led action. Take a moment now to play with this prayer-as-program before you move on. Repeat the prayer to yourself or ask yourself these questions:

Today, what am I clinging onto that I cannot change? And what can I change and courageously choose to do differently?

I suspect you too will experience clarity and agency as you name what you cannot change (and therefore need to let go of) and what you have agency over (and therefore can move into self-led action around).

That feeling

Agency, coupled with self-efficacy, feels divine. The moment we acknowledge that we have a choice – that we don't have to do what our old trauma-led patterns are telling us to do – is life-changing. It feels this way because as we let go of what we cannot change and move towards what we can, our body moves out of contraction and towards expansion. The choice and the sense of agency signals safety to our nervous system and reconnects us to our adult self. I witness this moment in sessions every day. A client comes in tense, triggered and in pain because their wounded parts and adaptations believe they have no control, agency or freedom. They are in the glue, unable to step back and see that there's a different way.

The different way is the new way of being and relating you've been integrating: signalling safety, moving into presence and curiosity, and reconnecting back to your adult self so you can see with perspective and compassion. In session, this is what we do – first bring more safety and curiosity, then acknowledge triggered parts that are whispering an old story and old beliefs that keep us trapped in autopilot. Then we connect to our adult perspective so we can move into self-led agency and action.

This feeling, as we unlock our agency and connect to our own power to create change, is everything. It's the hopeful, expansive energy of trauma healing. We need as much of this glorious feeling as we can get. In many ways it is the antidote to trauma, and it exists within you.

Beyond the four capacities

Trauma healing energy is unlocked as we integrate the four capacities. Other things can also move us into it. These *things* are pretty simple. So simple in fact that the clinical approach to trauma treatment often overlooks them. This happens for many reasons; one is that intellectual humans are predisposed to overcomplicating a problem. Trauma has been over-medicalised, so of course, trauma treatments are often over-medicalised.

Trauma healing requires us to see and bring resolution to our past pain. The moments from our past that felt terrifying and too much must now be felt safely and understood in an adult way. But we must also begin allowing ourselves to experience the things we've missed out on. Autopilot has moved us into disconnection and contraction. Healing is about moving into connection and expansion. To heal, we cannot myopically study our pain. We must also courageously learn to experience the opposite – joy, play, creativity, flow, connection, expansion.

To understand more about how we can apply this idea to facilitate healing, I spoke to Josh Dickson, a remarkable EMDR clinician and trauma specialist. He, like me, is trying to do things differently. Josh is the founder of Resurface, an organisation that runs trauma resolution retreats combining EMDR and surfing. Yes. Surfing. From the outside looking in, trauma resolution *surf* retreats appear niche. But the idea is born from Josh's time studying the benefits of positive psychology – the scientific study of why people flourish and thrive. Josh explained:

Positive psychology transforms trauma healing by shifting our focus beyond just managing symptoms to building real resilience and meaning. This matters because when we're dealing with trauma, we need both – healing what hurts and creating a foundation for growth. We weave this into treatment by helping people recognise their strengths, practise gratitude, and find purpose, all while honouring their healing journey.

There's a powerful evidence-based method behind the inclusion of surfing in Josh's model of trauma healing. Surfing, like any enjoyable activity we get absorbed in as we learn, moves us into *flow state*. Josh continued:

Flow state is fascinating because it's this sweet spot where you're completely absorbed in what you're doing. Time seems to fade away, and you're just fully present. It's incredibly powerful for healing because it creates a unique state in your brain and body where stress hormones drop, a cocktail of natural feel-good chemicals increase (dopamine, anandamide, endorphins, serotonin, oxytocin), and your nervous system finds this beautiful balance of being both calm and engaged. This gives your system a chance to experience safety while staying active, which helps create new patterns that contrast with the inactivity of trauma.

To find flow in everyday life, you don't need anything fancy. You might get lost in great conversation, or feel totally absorbed in drawing, while running or dancing, or working in your garden. The key is choosing something you enjoy that's challenging enough to keep you engaged but not so hard it causes too much frustration. Play works in similar ways, although it isn't necessarily challenging in the way flow is – both play and flow help you step out of self-consciousness, stay present, and naturally build confidence through enjoyment rather than pressure.

As I talked you through Capacity One, I explained that connection signals safety to the nervous system. I suggested walking in nature, listening to podcasts or giving your dog a cuddle, among other things, as ways to safely begin to move back into connection. I also explained that this sense of connection is born from practising anchoring and soothing as we do this. Because cuddling your dog while, say, angrily listing all the reasons you hate your boss does not constitute *connection*.

The concept of flow – the brain state we move into when we're absorbed in something we enjoy doing – expands the concept of healing through connection. I love it because it's so empowering, clear and directive. Flow is achieved in many ways. You don't have to go surfing, although knock yourself out if that's your bag. We move into flow state as we learn something we feel excited to learn, so we're completely present and engaged. I've witnessed clients transform as they integrated the four capacities while also starting a new creative hobby, increasing their sense of flow.

Ceramics, weight training, lino printing, cooking, yoga, silk painting, kayaking, horse riding, flamenco dancing, tai chi, life drawing, gardening and rock climbing are just a few of the activities I've seen *facilitate* trauma healing. A great many other creative, playful, expansive activities would also facilitate healing as we practise them with presence and passion. It's not about the specific activity you choose, but the state of flow we move into as we allow and embody these things. Flow state combines with an increased sense of agency (I have choice and can effect change) and self-efficacy (I can do this) to build resilience, move our nervous system out of trauma-led patterns and allow us to embody *that* feeling.

As a last word on this, I also need to point out that many of us (myself included) can use the concepts of flow, play and mastery to beat ourselves up. They can easily and quickly become something we *should* be doing, but are failing to do. These concepts, then, can trigger our *I'm getting it all wrong* or *I'm not doing enough* wounding. In response to a list of fun, light, playful activities, we subconsciously change the goal posts. A sense of not-enoughness, pressure and push replaces regulation, curiosity and a balanced adult perspective. Take a moment now to consider if this old wounding may have been activated by the ideas I'm talking about here. If this feels true for you, please hear this:

You are doing enough. You are moving into healing. Now may not be the best time for you start a new activity, and that's okay. Instead try to approach life with a little more of the *attitude* of flow and play. Cook dinner mindfully. Dance in your kitchen. Play with your dog. Small moments of flow and play are what we're looking for – don't let this concept derail your recovery and pull you back into old beliefs that are not true.

Adult perspective

Giving ourselves permission to lean into what feels good, what feels new and fun, is irritatingly painful for many. It goes against our programming. 'Start a new hobby that lights you up' is a simple directive, but certainly not an easy one. Those with unresolved childhood trauma are in various states of deprivation (page 80). We're also in various states of contraction and avoidance (page 122). We can find other people and social situations overwhelming and confusing (page 81). Protective parts are often so afraid of failure, we get stuck in freeze, so we struggle to move into action (page 129). Worse of all, it's likely that wounded parts of us do not believe they deserve good things (page 236). Our old trauma-led patterns make choosing, implementing and standing by this 'simple' action very difficult indeed. What may seem like a frivolous, delightful, easy action to take (say, a ceramics class) in reality is far from it.

The solution to the pain that can accompany these self-led actions is found in the first three capacities. To move into action around anything at all, be it ceramics, self-care or setting a boundary, we must:

- Hold ourselves through the discomfort by signalling safety and regulating
- Curiously observe our own reaction and response
- Unblend from parts with compassion
- Reconnect back to our adult self.

As we anchor back into our adult self we become able to give ourselves what we need. We give ourselves the corrective, supportive experience that will empower us into agency and action. The research of psychologist Albert Bandura into self-efficacy (belief that we can effect change) demonstrates that it's slowly built through mastery and adult verbal persuasion.[1] In other words, we develop self-belief as we learn a new thing, while also developing the skill of supporting ourselves through the learning.

Over time, as we increasingly anchor into our adult self, we practise encouraging ourselves through tough, uncomfortable moments with phrases like, 'You can do this.' We practise responding with compassion and an adult perspective when we make a mistake: 'It's okay, everyone makes mistakes – it's how we learn.' We hold the line when we sense we have the capacity to stretch: 'I know you're feeling anxious about going, but you can do it – let's give it a try.' We also notice when it really is too much for us, when it's no longer stretching us but stressing us and pushing our nervous system too far: 'This is too much for you today, let's go tomorrow instead.'

If this sounds like you're suddenly reading a parenting book, that's because you are. Here I'm talking about *reparenting*, because childhood trauma healing requires (yes, *requires*) us to learn how to become our own wise, loving parent. The balancing adult presence and voice of connection, calm, curiosity, compassion, reason and empowerment are deeply healing because they provide corrective experiences and allow us to move from contraction to release. They also help us increasingly move into agency and action.

Flow, play, creativity and mastery facilitate trauma healing, but moving into these kinds of self-led actions requires us to encourage and support ourselves, just as a parent would.

Authentic and aligned

We've gradually been building our understanding of self (see Diagram 6 on page 255 to get a sense of what I'm talking about). As we move through Capacity Four, we pull more concepts into our understanding of self: limits, wants, needs, values, authenticity and alignment.

Being in self – regulated, aware, adult – allows us to see, feel and connect to our limits, wants, needs and values. We come to know ourselves on a deeper level, becoming aware of these integral aspects of self. This is self-knowing, and over time, this self-knowing directs the action we take. We move from trauma-led action, where our wounding and protective adaptations unconsciously direct our action, to self-led action, where our adult self consciously directs our choices and actions. Over time we feel, and are increasingly authentic and in alignment with, an anchored sense of self.

To help you understand what I mean, I want to tell you about one of my wonderful clients, Carrie. Carrie had an alcoholic father and a mother who experienced extreme emotional highs and lows (recently diagnosed with bipolar). Carrie trod the path many take in response to this kind of upbringing. She developed an eating disorder and moved into rigid patterns of control around her appearance and schoolwork. Carrie then married into a highly dysfunctional, authoritarian family system. She was drawn to the family because the rigidity and strict rules felt like the antidote to the chaos she was raised in. Carrie moulded herself into the daughter-in-law they expected her to be, and in doing so further disconnected from her agency and her authentic self.

The family used micro-aggressions and covert control to communicate their expectations about how Carrie should behave. When she said what she really thought or stated a preference outside the narrow bounds of these expectations, she was subtly punished and rejected. After ten years of this, and after a consciousness-piercing moment of her own, Carrie got in touch with me.

Carrie was nervous, unsure and triggered. She had lost touch with herself and reality – unsure how she felt, what she thought, what was right and wrong, what she wanted and what she needed. Of course this was the space Carrie was in – she'd been told what to think and feel for a decade.

In sessions now, fourteen months on, Carrie is funny, grounded and connected to her adult self. She knows what she wants and needs. She understands where her limits are and has a sense of her own values.

Carrie's transformation is remarkable and can only be credited to her and the self-led action she's taken. Yes, Carrie and I have been working together for over a year. I have been a safe place for her to land, this is true. But Carrie's healing was born from moments in her life when she courageously took action that aligned with her deepening sense of self.

As Carrie integrated capacities One, Two and Three, she reconnected to her adult self. As this anchored connection deepened, Carrie came to know herself, and over time, was able to take action that felt fully aligned with self.

To begin with, this was as simple as saying 'no thank you' when she was offered a cup of tea she didn't want to drink. Before this work, the question, 'Do you want a cup of tea?' would trigger Carrie. She'd be flooded with an old wounding – 'I'm getting it all wrong' – and a protective fawn part would swoop in, telling her to comply and say yes. Her life consisted of a million moments of this trauma-led response pattern – panic and comply. Recovery and healing came as Carrie practised first soothing the part of her that panicked, so she was able to begin to reconnect to her regulated adult self. Once there was more regu-lation and connection, Carrie was eventually able to *feel* her limits and wants (her no or yes). Once she could feel what she did and didn't want, Carrie then practised voicing it – first to neutral others outside of the family, and then slowly within the family.

Over the past year, Carrie's relationship with her husband's family has deteriorated. Now she's no longer adhering to the role she was required to fill, she's less liked. This has been profoundly upsetting for Carrie. At various points she's had to stop and ask herself, 'Is this worth it?' *Yes* is the resounding answer she hears back. She chooses being disliked over dysregulation, self-abandonment, self-blame, self-hate, control and fawning.

I knew we'd got there when in a session Carrie said to me: 'I'm not going to Sunday lunch – I can't sit around in all the passive aggression. I need a break. I'm going to the cinema with a friend instead. I love going to the movies.'

This is self-led, aligned action. Carrie was clear about her limits, able to uphold them, and aware of her own preferences and able to act on them. The action Carrie chose to take isn't objectively right or wrong. Had she decided to go to the lunch with the same level of awareness and conviction this too would have been a win. It's not about the choice we make, it's about where it's coming from. It's about becoming able to make a self-led choice rather than a trauma-led one. It's about self-knowing, self-acceptance, self-agency and self-efficacy. These are the gifts of recovery and trauma healing.

Limits

Limits are boundaries – they're the things we do to keep ourselves comfortable, safe, regulated, healing and in self. As we increasingly live in connection with our body, and with awareness of our window of tolerance, we become able to feel where our limits are. Pushing through, performing and operating from a dysregulated part becomes increasingly unappealing, because we can feel just how damaging this way of being is to our body. It feels increasingly inauthentic and misaligned. A beautiful new desire to stay within our window of tolerance, operating from the green zone and in connection with our adult self, means we feel increasingly compelled to state and uphold our limits. We can feel, and then act on, our embodied 'no'. Examples of limits:

- Saying 'no' to an invite
- Asking a family member to communicate without shouting
- Telling a friend you can only speak on the phone for ten minutes
- Saying 'no' to a colleague who wants you to attend a meeting during your lunch break
- Asking a colleague not to message after work hours.

Trauma healing requires us to put down boundaries and limits. Although this is uncomfortable initially, as we practise, it becomes easier. Remember psychologist Ingrid Clayton's words of wisdom: breaking these patterns can hurt, but the healing comes as we learn to hold ourselves through the discomfort (page 140).

In the moment, any signs that you're going into the orange or red zone (page 172) indicate that you may need to set a limit. Ideally though, and as Carrie did, we set the limit *before* we enter the orange or red zone. This is possible over time as we increasingly connect to reality *and* make choices that reflect our adult perspective. Just as a wise, loving parent does, we learn to set the boundaries and limits that best support our wellbeing so we don't move past our 'too much' line (page 144).

From a place of regulation and anchored self, consider for a moment what feels too much for you (and your wounded/ protective parts) at the moment. Think about moments in the day that routinely feel stressful or overwhelming. Think about moments in relationships that are routinely pushing you into a triggered reaction. Think also about future situations that are already provoking an intense internal reaction. Now consider ways you can most easily implement some limits and boundaries to create more comfort and ease in your life (and therefore in your nervous system).

Wants

Wants are preferences – the things we like, love, desire and enjoy. As we move out of unconscious autopilot, we increasingly live in conscious connection with the present moment and our body. This reconnection doesn't bring with it a clear list of likes and dislikes, but it does move us into exploration. As we anchor into self and unlock our agency and self-efficacy, we become able to explore what we want, what we like and what we enjoy in a flexible, light-hearted way. Some examples of wants, likes and preferences are:

- I enjoy hot showers.
- I prefer to drink tea, not coffee, first thing in the morning.
- I love listening to funny political podcasts.
- I like eating healthy food.
- I love Marvel movies.
- I prefer winter clothing to summer clothing.

I won't give more example as wants, likes and preferences are a pretty easy category to get our heads around. We can connect to our wants, likes and preferences at any time. We can also connect to them in the moment when we're faced with a choice. To do either, we first self-regulate and then move into curiosity to ask ourselves what we want, like or prefer. This could sound like:

- What do I want right now?
- What would I like to do today?
- Which would I prefer today?

I found exploring my wants, likes and preferences really hard. I had been so disconnected from my body during my teens and twenties that understanding what I wanted felt very challenging. But the examples I gave above, on page 287, are all my own likes and preferences. I'm aware there's nothing mind-blowingly interesting in this little list, but being able to state my preferences so clearly means a lot to me after years of morphing and disconnecting. If you feel stumped by this work, remind yourself that this is a process of exploration. Give yourself permission not to know and allow yourself to make a light-hearted choice, which can sound like, 'I'm not sure – so I'll choose this one.' Over time as you explore, you'll get a sense of what you like and prefer.

Needs

Needs are more essential – the things we require to function and thrive. Reconnection to our needs feels uncomfortable for those who have tried to deny their own needs as a way of coping. This protective adaptation/part is very common – we push away our own innate human needs as a way to try and remain in connection with another human. We are our lowest priority, often preferring to serve everyone else's needs rather than state our own. Reconnecting to our body, our emotions and our adult self reconnects us to our innate physiological and emotional needs. Once we can feel and sense them, we practise taking self-led action to meet our needs. Some examples of needs are:

- Sleep
- Security
- Friendship

- Intimacy
- Recognition
- Personal growth.

You might have heard of 'Maslow's hierarchy of needs', designed by the psychologist Abraham Maslow. This system groups needs into physiological needs like sleep, safety needs such as security, love and belonging needs such as friendship, esteem needs such as recognition and self-actualisation needs such as personal growth.

Connecting to our needs is done in the moment. It's about slowing down and doing what you've been practising – regulating and then moving into conscious awareness and curious observation. Once we're in connection we simply ask ourselves: what do I need, right now?

Values

Values are things that are important to us. Knowing our values is helpful, because they can direct our choices and the action we take. For example, considering whether a specific decision is aligned with our values helps us sense whether we're moving in a direction that will feel good and comfortable. Values change over time, which is why it's helpful to reflect on our current values. This is all the more important for those who've been stuck in trauma-led autopilot and disconnected from our adult self and values. Some examples of values are:

- Authenticity
- Forgiveness
- Loyalty

- Courage
- Adventurousness
- Accountability
- Commitment
- Compassion
- Originality
- Equality
- Kindness.

To begin to get a sense of your own values, ask yourself these questions when you're regulated and anchored into self:

- What's important to me and why?
- What do I respect and appreciate in other people and why?
- What are my priorities and why?

Try to hold this exercise lightly – there are no right or wrong answers. Your values will be present in your 'why'. For example, if you wrote, 'My friends are important to me because of the laughter and joy they bring into my life,' it's likely that joy is one of your values. If you wrote, 'My work is important to me because it gives me a sense of fulfilment,' it's likely that fulfilment is one of your values. And if you wrote, 'Exercise is a priority for me because it enhances my sense of wellbeing,' it's likely that wellbeing is one of your values.

To help you turn your 'why' into a list of values, review the list of common values in Appendix E. Once you've got a sense of your values, find the six that are the most important to you. These are your core values.

Being aware of our values doesn't mean we're automatically going to start operating from them, but it does give us useful information to consider as we make decisions and design our life. And, just as with limits, wants and needs, stating and knowing our values can feel deeply satisfying and important after years of disconnection.

Being in self (regulated, aware and adult) allows us to connect to these fundamental aspects of who we are. For many, this work is the first time they've consciously become aware of these aspects of self. Before this reconnection to the body and the self, wounding and protective parts tend to direct our choices and decisions. Without conscious awareness, trauma rather than self was leading life. This leads many to wake up one day realising they feel disconnected and lacking authenticity. We realise our lives don't feel authentically ours or aligned with who we really are. Trauma healing moves us into authenticity. As we feel incrementally safer, we become able to see our patterns, emotions, parts, wounding and adaptations. But we also become able to see, feel, own and stand by our preferences, limits and values. From this self-connection, and as we integrate the other three capacities, we can start creating the life we want and need.

Positive agitation

The title of this section – positive agitation – is taken from a conversation I had with Calum Morrison – the founder and CEO of The Extraordinary Adventure Club (EAC). Calum and his team lean into the whole doing things differently philosophy: they curate unusual experiences, meticulously designed to bring about self-reconnection, change and growth in a client.

As an example of the kind of extraordinary adventures he curates, Calum told me about a high-profile client whose every outfit, comment, weight fluctuation and private life were subject to scrutiny. So much so that she withdrew from public life, hiding in her house, becoming more and more isolated and anxious. He explained:

We utilised her love of horses and childhood dream of competing in a rodeo as a thread to pull her out of her self-imposed exile. She participated in a large rodeo in South America, competing in a barrel race in front of a crowd of thousands. She was schooled prior to the race by the previous Rodeo Queen and came second. We choreographed the event to ensure she was interviewed by the Ringmaster and spoke in front of a crowd of thousands. The change was astonishing.

Calum continued:

It's absolutely possible to create meaningful, deep change outside of the therapy room. Though one doesn't preclude the other. Both modalities can be aligned in mutually supporting ways to effect meaningful change.

We achieve this change through intentional theatre – positively agitating those we work with, dislocating their expectations through a curated interplay between the key elements of content, tempo and sequence.

Calum went on to unpack this idea of positive agitation:

We disconnect clients from the framework that holds them in a particular place or way of thinking, in order to reconnect them with themselves. We remove watches and phones and any other distractions that act as anchor points for them to cling to. Our clients never know where they're going or the itinerary of the program, they let go of this notion of control and are forced to focus on being in the moment. Too little of modern life is raw and free-flowing, too much is carefully directed and constrained.

Elements of physical, emotional and mental hardship precede transformation. This transformation is not a passive act but an active endeavour. In order to change behaviours and develop better thinking, the process requires consistency and commitment. It's about developing resilience, self-sufficiency and personal responsibility. We build skills and create confidence through the incremental accumulation of competence.

Finally, I asked Calum how those of us who aren't on one of his extraordinary adventures can apply aspects of his approach to create change in this extraordinary way. He replied:

Move outside your normal environment. Change the framework. Remove your phone and take off your watch. Move your body. Go for a walk. Find a place where you won't be disturbed. Raise awareness through curiosity and notice things that are so often overlooked. Sit holding an intention, without distraction. Slow your breathing. It is incremental consistency that creates significant and lasting change, not one event. There are no shortcuts or hacks. It takes patience and practice.

Calum and his team take people out of the systems and frameworks that are maintaining the problem. They remove people from environments, jobs, people and cues that trigger old, unhelpful adaptations. In doing so, they afford their clients a freedom to explore and reconnect to who they are underneath the patterning and the autopilot.

This idea can be pulled into the work you're doing as you integrate Capacity Four. Take space, literally, from the systems you're locked into. Curate your own adventure and challenge, leave your old way of being at home, and as you move out of autopilot you'll get a deeper sense of who you truly are, and what you truly want, value and need.

From reacting to creating

As we increasingly operate from self, agency and self-belief build, and we become increasingly able to choose. We go from having little choice over how we react, what we say, how we feel and behave, to having increasing choice about these things. We become able to choose how we show up in the world, how we respond and the action we choose to take.

I've already mentioned my client Rose to you – the emergency nurse who can now regulate and remain connected to her adult self during emergency resuscitations. Last week, Rose said: 'Because I'm no longer reacting, I'm able to create the life experience I want.' She went on to describe how she now approaches her day with a new, empowered sense of freedom and choice. 'As I go into situations I ask myself: How do I want to experience this? What do I, as my present adult self, want this to feel like?'

Such agency and action were not available to Rose before she started healing and integrating the four capacities. She was on autopilot. Now, and for the first time in her life, she's consciously creating the life she wants: choosing who she wants to be with, choosing what she says and how she approaches situations.

This glorious new sense of agency that's now available to Rose is a direct outcome of the daily self-led actions she took:

- Learn how to regulate and signal safety to her nervous system.
- Learn how to move into curious observation and greater awareness.
- Learn how to separate from and compassionately receive her younger parts, so she could operate from her adult self.
- Learn to connect to her own agency and then take authentic, aligned self-led action in the world around her.

Rose's experience emphasises the power of the self-led approach and of trauma healing generally. We all want and deserve to move through life with a sense of freedom, empowerment and choice. As we see and interrupt our trauma-led patterns we unlock our agency and ability to create real, aligned, authentic change in our lives.

Play with this idea today. As you move through the day, ask yourself, just as Rose did: 'How do I want to experience this? What do I, as my present adult self, want this to feel like?'

Like Rose, you can also apply these questions to the future by asking yourself: 'What do I want to be experiencing in five years' time? From a place of adult self, what do I want my life to look and feel like five years from now?'

These questions will reconnect you to your agency and choice, to your limits, values, wants and needs, so you can have a different, healing experience. And so you can begin to create from a place of self-led agency, rather than react from autopilot.

Self-led inaction

The whole premise of this book is that we heal as we gently and appropriately begin to take self-led action. Although this premise remains, I also need to highlight that choosing to do nothing – to pause, wait for more information, curiously observe and allow life to unfold – constitutes *action*. There's a huge difference between this (consciously choosing to do nothing) and unconsciously avoiding and resisting action.

Anchored, regulated self-led action interrupts old trauma patterns, allows us to release, and soothes our wounding and protective parts. Choosing to do nothing from a place of self has the same effect. So before you dive into this new, self-led way of living, remember that self-led inaction is, in fact, action.

Self-acceptance

I want to close this chapter with some words from my conversation with Dr Brad Reedy, a therapist, author and founder of the Finding You therapy programs. His therapeutic approach is designed to create deep transformation and change by helping clients connect to and accept who they truly are. During our time together, Brad explained to me why he puts authenticity and self-acceptance at the centre of his therapeutic approach:

> [The therapist and founder of person-centred therapy] Carl Rogers says that "it's only when I accept myself that I can change." To find one's truth, you have to get to a place where it's okay to be who you are. Because what blocks us from this is our sense that the feelings, the thoughts, the urges, the impulses that are in us are wrong, immature or too sensitive. Our parents and teachers said that they were out of place – we've been taught that they were wrong.
>
> As my own therapist says: if I can allow you to be your horrible rotten self in therapy and I can love

your horrible rotten self, then you'll start to love who you are. From that authentic connection with yourself, your expression in the universe will be love. It'll be love because you won't be fighting to be right, to be good, to be proper. You'll just be you. And that is so much better than being right and good.

I love what James Hollis says, that the biggest barrier to getting what we want in our lives is who we have become up to this point. And that is a result of our conditioning, of our teaching, of our culture, of our situation, of our context. Basically, it has told us who we should be, who's the good person to be, what good people do. This is what white people do, this is what black people do, this is what girls do, this is what boys do, and we believe that stuff because we have no other choice as little people. Until you realise that all the things that you've been taught that would make you happy didn't make you happy, and then you start to seek something different.

Brad seeks to help his clients feel safe enough to move through resistance, shame, fear, wounding and protective adaptations, so they can accept every part of themselves and move into authentic self-led living. Every time you pause, move out of unconscious autopilot and connect to reality you meet yourself authentically. Every time you notice fear and anger, observe your worries, unblend or see and validate parts, you meet yourself authentically. Every time you pause, regulate, and from a place of self, consider what you want or need, you meet yourself authentically. As you do this alongside signalling safety, regulation and compassion, you will move into self-acceptance and you will heal.

Stay on your own side

Reparenting – learning to be that voice of reason and compassion – is necessary to support ourselves as we start to make different, new choices in life. But it's also necessary because other people are likely to have opinions about our new way of being and living. Or if they don't, we might project one (most likely an opinion that belongs to one of our own protector parts) onto them.

So reparenting is also about learning to stay on our own side. Just as a parent would, we do not abandon ourselves. We do this as we learn to hold ourselves, our wants, our needs, our choices, our opinions and our mistakes, in a new, regulated way. We practise moving back into self-connection as we feel the younger parts of us react from fear. We hold our parts' hands instead of throwing them (and ourselves) under the bus. Alongside compassion (rather than criticism) and curiosity (rather than judgement), and just as a parent would, we learn to hold a balanced, level-headed, adult perspective (rather than abandoning, persecuting, catastrophising, denying, collapsing, defending, despairing or blaming).

I feel compelled to point this out because I haven't yet had a client for whom this isn't relevant. During an uncomfortable moment in a relational dynamic, we're prone to disconnect from self and move into protective parts that self-blame, self-hate, give up, collapse, pander, judge and criticise us. We do this unconsciously to try and remain safe. During these triggering moments, we need to find our way back to our adult self so we can continue to take aligned, self-led action rather than moving back into trauma-led action.

This takes practice. It's okay if this seems wildly out of reach right now. The capacities you're integrating – signalling safety, curiously observing your reaction, separating from parts, reconnecting back to your adult self and acknowledging your agency – are how we achieve this remarkable, life-changing feat. So, again, there's nothing new here – integrate the four capacities and you'll become increasingly able to stay on your own side, and therefore increasingly able to take action that feels aligned with who you are and what you want.

Make the call

In Chapter Three: The consequences I explained that childhood trauma predisposes us to self-sufficiency (page 71). For a very long time I thought healing meant 'being able to do everything on my own'. The penny-drop moment came as I realised that at the top of the mountain, we're able to *make the call*.

We all struggle to be our own wise, loving adult at times. There are times we cannot be our own source of 'adult verbal persuasion', when we cannot encourage and cheerlead for ourselves, when we cannot hold our mistakes with compassion, when we cannot stay on our own side. These moments are not a sign you're broken. They simply prove you are human. All humans need other humans to encourage, cheerlead, love and support them. When you struggle to do this for yourself, make the call. Reach out to someone you trust, tell them what you need and allow them to support you.

If this idea stings because you look around and see no-one you can call, you're not alone. This is a common realisation for those with unresolved childhood trauma. As we wake up and reconnect back to the present moment and ourselves, many of us realise that our relationships struggle to hold the most vulnerable parts of us. Over time, you may find that some of these relationships can change as you change. But if not, slowly start to find other soft places to land (page 161).

Chapter Ten

The reality of the mountain top

In all honesty, I've said much of what needs saying. You don't need more theory, more explanations, more words about how to heal your trauma. You've made it this far, so you understand the essence of my argument: therapy alone cannot heal trauma, and therefore cannot heal the plethora of problems and issues trauma creates, but therapy coupled with self-led action to integrate the four capacities of healing will create deep and lasting healing. I hope this approach resonates with you, inspires you and moves you into deep and lasting change.

This chapter is primarily about the reality of the mountain top you're making your way to. Towards the end of the chapter, I also include practical, real-life information on the nitty gritty of trauma healing (for example, on different modalities and residential centres).

The mountain top

Before I talk about the reality of the mountain top – the often unexpected aspects of trauma healing, change and growth – I want to clearly explain what the mountain top looks and feels like. So, here are 25 beautiful signs that you're healing trauma, regulating your nervous system and creating real change:

1. You feel safer in your body.
2. You feel connected to your body, your emotions, your inner world.
3. You can hold a dual perspective.*
4. You feel more emotionally and mentally present with others and in life.
5. You feel more open to relationships and being around other people.
6. Your highs and lows feel less extreme.
7. You experience less hypervigilance.
8. You have more energy and motivation.
9. Your physical health improves.
10. You feel less sensitive to stimulation.
11. You feel less triggered.
12. You feel you have to avoid triggers less often.
13. You feel an anchored sense of self and know who you are.
14. You trust your own perspective, reality and intuition.
15. You feel connected to your sense of self even during emotional fluctuations.
16. You know you can cope in a healthy way – that you're okay.

---

* In trauma healing, being able to hold a dual perspective means we can be aware of two things at once. Such as feeling grateful while also being aware of feelings of grief, or feeling connected to your body whilst also listening to another speak.

17. You can unblend from and soothe parts of yourself.
18. You feel more curious about yourself and others.
19. You feel more compassion.
20. You feel comfortable with emotional intimacy.
21. You feel comfortable with physical intimacy and touch.
22. You feel more open, playful and joyful.
23. You can ask for help and support when you need it.
24. You live with a greater sense of authenticity and alignment.
25. You know, and can act on, your limits and preferences.

Maybe that was the most satisfying, joy-filled list I've ever compiled – certainly more satisfying than the to-do lists I'm usually compiling. What a delight it is to think of all the healing and growth I've witnessed in others over the years and experienced myself. This list is not unattainable or unrealistic. The opposite is actually true – it's possible, very possible, to experience every single one of the 25 outcomes. This list describes my own internal and external experience of life today. But there was a time that I experienced the reverse of every single one of these 25 signs. I felt unsafe in my body, was profoundly disconnected from it, my emotions and my inner world (and was triggered anytime I went anywhere near them), had no idea what a dual perspective was, let alone the capacity to hold one, and was completely lost in my own pain and autopilot, rather than being present emotionally and mentally. Literally every single sign was a mystery to me.

If this is where you're at – if you're also operating from the reverse list, as I was – exhale. You're supposed to start in the forest at the bottom of the mountain. These 25 signs of healing will slowly unfurl in your mind, body, sense of self and life. It takes time, for some years, but it will come. One day, you will look at this list and you will smile because you will know you're at the top of the mountain.

The reality of being human

Okay, real talk. As I've mentioned many times, trauma healing is about anchoring into reality. I'm all for travelling hopefully – in fact, hope is essential – but we can be hopeful, even joyful and playful, whilst being in reality, rather than in trauma and denial. Over the years, we've disconnected from the reality of our emotions, self-concept, beliefs, bodies, relationships, purpose, desires, preferences and limits. As we heal, we reconnect to these things. Our reality, and therefore our truth and authenticity, come back into focus.

Reality, then, is what we're shooting for here, and as the word implies, it's not always . . . fun. In my twenties, for example, as I anchored into reality I had to acknowledge that I ate (or didn't eat) compulsively as a way to cope. In my thirties, reality came crashing into conscious awareness as I understood that the stress and trauma I was operating from was harming my body. I've mentioned these moments of pain piercing conscious awareness before (page 44), so I won't belabour the point.

Here, in this final chapter, I'm more interested in the reality of how if feels to stand at the top of the mountain than the painful moments of awareness that inevitably accompany our journey to the top. Because standing at the top of the mountain, as you will, doesn't only consist of those 25 signs. It also consists of feeling uncomfortable feelings, grief and self-doubt, among other things. Sounds fun, right? Okay, fun might be a stretch, but all I've done here is name some of the less sparkly aspects of being human.

The reality of being human is, at times, messy, and seems very far from those 25 signs of recovery. But, given that reality is the goal, we're going to need to aim for (or at least accept) the less than perfect parts of being human. There's a lot of imperfect humanness I could cover here, of course. But I'm going to focus on the things I witness clients struggle with the most: not having a playbook, feeling feelings, appropriate grief and anger, self-doubt and our evolution.

No playbook

First up, let's talk about the fact that none of us have a playbook for living life at the top of mountain. We know what we do when we're in our trauma, in the forest at the bottom of the mountain, but we don't know how to do life at the top.

The neural map we have been using to navigate life – which consists of trauma patterning and survival states – is obsolete. We're in the process of creating a new one. I know I've mentioned this before in the book: the process of interrupting old patterns and laying down new ones is what this whole self-led healing thing is about. But here, I want to highlight that although this sounds expansive and exciting (and in many ways, it is), it requires us to get comfortable living life without a playbook for a while.

'I don't know what I'm doing here,' 'I'm totally winging it,' 'I feel like I'm walking off the edge of a cliff,' and 'I feel like I'm running in the dark,' are all phrases clients have recently used to described the exquisite pain that accompanies mountain-top life.

What I need you to know is that this feeling – this expansive, exciting, terrifying feeling – is not a sign that there's anything wrong. In fact, this feeling is a sign that everything is very right indeed.

I'm not advocating for you to live the rest of your life feeling as if you're walking off a cliff. That would be quite an intense, bizarre state to permanently exist in. But I do want you to know that this feeling is largely the result of having a sudden awareness that you have no playbook – no habitual patterning – to fall back on. Theoretically it's good, of course, to no longer move into survival as a way to cope and navigate relationships. But survival – fight, flight, freeze, fawn and collapse – supplied us with a strong, automatic rulebook for life. As you integrate the four capacities and do your trauma work, you relinquish this rulebook. And as theoretically divine as this sounds, in reality it's fucking terrifying.

I hope you'll remember my words here when this odd, slightly out of control, exhilarating feeling hits you. Because you'll wonder: Is this a sign I'm unwell and damaged? Am I safe? Am I getting things wrong? Does anyone else feel this way?

Hear me when I say – all is well. You are at the top of the mountain. You are safe.

Feeling

Trauma prevents us from feeling uncomfortable feelings, so, of course, trauma healing involves feeling those feelings. I've explained this before – the feelings you've been avoiding, which stem from your past and your wounding, need to slowly and gently be allowed and experienced. We achieve this through pendulation – dipping in and out of the discomfort – gradually building tolerance.

The interesting thing about trauma healing is that as we unfold the survival adaptations and reconnect to our adult self and our bodies, and as our nervous system moves us out of contraction and protection, we feel *more*. Just this week a client, Laura, arrived to the session saying she was extremely emotional. Laura told me, 'I'm crying so often, which is so unlike me. I'm not sobbing, just welling-up constantly at the smallest things.'

'And how is that for you?' I asked.

'I love it,' she replied. She continued, 'It's so unlike me – I'm usually so buttoned-up, so it feels important and different to be so in touch with sadness and joy.'

Self-led healing, and all trauma work, allows emotions to follow the bell curve – that beautiful crescendo, peak and discharge of emotion-as-energy that comes as we move through life in a connected way. Crying spontaneously, feeling a swell of love, sadness, joy or grief in our chest, or experiencing appropriate anger, are all parts of life lived at the top of the mountain.

Grief, sadness, regret, resentment and anger

As we feel safer in our bodies, our awareness expands – we can see and feel *more*. The expansion of awareness leads the self-led action we take to create a new way of being and relating. This all sounds rather lovely and powerful, doesn't it? And it is. Trauma healing is an expansive process – it's not all about pain. My official position on trauma and trauma healing is that we do not have to be afraid of it. We can understand it, we can heal and we can grow from it. As true as this is, it's also true that as our awareness expands, we see a reality that doesn't feel very expansive at all. Of course, as we do our trauma work we become aware of and process our trauma — the moments, the relationships, the beliefs, the protective adaptations, the wounding, the survival states and the patterning that are strewn through our past. This is the nature of what we're doing here. The centre of the work, which we slowly and respectfully move towards as we gradually increase our tolerance, is all this old stuff.

Over time, as we integrate the capacities, we come to see things clearly and with an adult perspective. And with this adult perspective come waves of appropriate disbelief, anger, grief, sadness, resentment or a sense of loss or regret. The sense of anguish and grief that may accompany a realisation that, say, we were not loved the way we deserved to be, is deeply painful. It's also appropriate and important to allow oneself to feel these things.

The reality of the mountain top is that along with the beauty of seeing yourself and your life clearly and as an anchored adult, you will inevitably understand how much you have been hurt. You may feel anger, sadness and grief on behalf of your child self. You may feel these things intensely at times. Know that this is okay, appropriate and part of your healing.

These feelings need to be experienced, felt and mobilised – they need to be allowed to move and flow. They need to be witnessed by you (your adult self) and, most likely, by another adult too.

Remember all you have learned here. The Principles of Self-led Integration and the four capacities will hold you through this. Signal safety, pendulate in and out of the pain, find support and soft places to land, move into presence, anchor into your compassion and perspective and acknowledge your agency so you can move into action.

Self-doubt

Self-trust takes time to build. Over time, we come to trust our nervous system's capacity to regulate. We come to trust our awareness and perspective. We also come to trust our capacity to respond to ourselves with compassion and the direction our self-led action takes us. These new things – this new way of being – initially feel unreliable. In large part that's because at the beginning of this journey they *are* unreliable. The capacities and the principles feel slippery and inconsistent, because they are. Our new sense of self – our connection to our body and our anchored adult perspective – feels unstable. So of course there's self-doubt: Can I hold myself through this? Am I well? Am I seeing things clearly? Am I getting this wrong? Am I allowed to set a boundary? Am I setting the right boundary? Can I have a new kind of relationship? Can I make the right choice? Am I making good choices? Am I getting it all wrong?

The fact of the matter is that the part of us that believes and fears we're getting everything wrong is deeply triggered by the healing process we're undertaking. This part of us is activated and in fear around the newness and the trajectory of the changes. It questions everything. It undermines everything. It *is* our self-doubt.

The reality of the mountain top is that our parts are up there with us. And this part – the getting it wrong part – will be activated by the very fact you're stood up there! Like all your parts, its activation and presence lets you know it needs to be seen, heard and understood. It needs compassion. It needs a strong, wise adult to remind it: 'I see you, I know you're afraid of getting it all wrong, but all is well, you're safe.' As you integrate the capacities, you'll increasingly be able to do this for yourself. But there may be times when you need another strong, wise adult to bring this anchored reassurance to this part of you.

As a final thought on self-doubt, I want to add that our propensity to doubt ourselves and our perspective seems to be directly proportional to the amount of time spent in childhood knowing there was something terribly wrong, but being told we were imagining things, being too sensitive, making it up or overreacting.

I've noticed that now, when people use the term gaslighting, they usually caveat it with, 'Sorry to use this term, I know it's so overused.' I'm particularly aware of this when clients who were so very clearly gaslit in childhood to an extreme and abusive level apologise for using the term.

In case you've been living under a rock and haven't heard of the term, gaslighting is the psychological manipulation of someone into questioning their own sanity or powers of reasoning.

Childhood trauma always involves confusion and mistrust in our own perspective. This is the nature of relational trauma and why it feels so messy. We have a sense that all is not okay, but lack the power of adult reason and objectivity to see things as they truly are. Doubting our own perspective and instinct, then, is something all of us need to acknowledge and heal from. But there are some who experienced this to an extreme level. They were gaslit as children – being explicitly told that abhorrent, abusive behaviour was normal, okay or warranted.

If you experienced this kind of psychological manipulation, what I've said is likely to resonate. It will provoke a feeling or a part, it may trigger a reaction that floods your system. If so, pause. Signal safety, respond to the parts with compassion and perspective.

No matter the level of self-doubt that our childhood contained, self-trust takes time to build and integrate. Yes, for some it takes longer than others, but the process of rebuilding is the same. We slowly integrate this essential characteristic as we integrate the four capacities and apply the principles. Over time, it develops as our sense of self becomes solid and reliable, as we see and feel that we can trust our perspective and as we see that life moves into alignment when we take self-led action. Healing the parts that doubt or the parts that have been gaslit cannot be rushed. But slowly, as we take self-led action internally and in life, we create a new kind of trust in ourselves and the way of being we have developed.

Other people

In the final chapter of my first book, *You're Not Broken*, I describe the problem that is other people's reactions to the changes that happen as a result of trauma healing. I don't like to repeat myself, but I can't let you head off without first giving you the same warning.

Trauma locks us into roles, parts, adaptations and states. This is the autopilot we've talked about. Those who live with you, who love you, who work with you, know you and spend time with you, are used to this autopilot version of you. They're used to the energy you bring and the roles you occupy. They're used to, say, you overworking and overdoing, to you having few boundaries and not saying no. They're used to the people-pleasing, the perfectionism, the self-doubt and the balance of power in the relationship.

You're locked into set, predictable dynamics with those around you. You move into, say, the helpless role, and your partner immediately moves into rescuer mode. Or perhaps the reverse of this is relevant for you. Or maybe your highly critical part activates a defensive part in your best friend. Parts activate parts and over time the positions we adopt in relationships become entrenched.

Changing these dynamics, showing up regulated and authentic rather than in autopilot is an essential part of healing. But it's also very challenging for those around us. Even if they don't like the status quo, they are used to the way we are. Many of our adaptations may even serve them in some way – if so, those around us will experience subconscious resistance as we move out of them.

Trauma healing is most greatly felt in our relationships, but not all relationships will readily expand to meet our changes. People may resist, grow angry, criticise, disconnect, shut down or panic as they see and feel us embrace a new way of being. This can be extremely painful and move us right back into self-doubt. We will find ourselves asking: Am I doing the right thing? Am I allowed to change? Should I continue up the mountain? Yes, unreservedly *yes* is the answer to these questions.

We can give those around us space and time, and we can be compassionate and curious about their experience, but we nevertheless continue our journey of self-connection and self-regulation. After a potentially bumpy period of adjustment, some relationships will expand and grow with you. These relationships will deepen as a result. Your healing and authenticity will give them permission to step out of their prescribed roles, and you will flourish together.

It's also true that some relationships will not be able to expand as you do. This has certainly been the case for me. As I reconnected to myself, I realised that I could not be fully well, fully regulated and fully authentically myself if I remained in certain relationships. So, after a long time spent painfully moving in and out of awareness and acceptance, slowly building tolerance, I took action to move out of these relationships. I chose myself. It was hard *and* it was important, empowering and authentic.

I dearly hope those you love can hold, accept and love you through the journey you're on. But, if they cannot, I hope you choose you over a life spent in survival and autopilot.

Apple Cider Vinegar

I recently watched *Apple Cider Vinegar* on Netflix. Maybe you've seen it? It's an uncomfortable watch, so I don't recommend it if you're not in a good place.

It's based on the true story of an Australian woman called Belle Gibson, who develops a healthy eating app marketed to people who are unwell. She claims to have healed a brain tumour simply by changing her diet. Her story and message are alluring, particularly for those undergoing painful medical treatment.

The implication by the end of the series, is that Belle is mentally unwell, desperate for attention and deeply traumatised. Because of her wounding, Belle fakes an illness that she then claims to have miraculously healed. As a result, people are harmed – walking away completely from mainstream medical advice and instead opting for an alternative treatment (i.e. juicing).

The program is pretty damning about alternative approaches to healing. If you're a sceptic, you'll love it. If you enjoy moving out of the mainstream as I do, it's confronting.

For me, it provoked an important recognition. In this book, I'm giving advice about supporting the healing of trauma, which I'm qualified to do. But also, without necessarily having set out to, I'm talking about supporting the healing of the body.

I claim that trauma contributes to many physiological illnesses (page 97). I claim that trauma healing is necessary for physical healing (page 100). I claim that visualising myself well (page 177) has facilitated wellness through nervous system regulation. Many claims, right.

What I propose in this book is theoretically sound and evidence-based. But it isn't the full picture.

So, before you head off and while I still have your attention, I want to be clear with you: I didn't *only* do my trauma work to integrate the four capacities. I did these things, yes, but I also:

- Took, and still take, medication
- Go to neurology appointments
- Follow an evidence-based MS diet
- Take supplements that support nervous system health.

I believe that I have much to gain from the medical advances that have taken place in the past two decades. Although, I do not blindly trust. I look at the research. I speak to others, listening to their opinions with curiosity so I can hear what they say without dismissing or pandering. I check in with my instinct before I take the medical advice I'm being given.

I take my time, and remain aware of my own agency and adult perspective, before I make a choice and act.

The choices I've outlined above are my own. They are not objectively right or wrong. They reflect my own preferences, instinct, knowledge, culture, privilege, access to healthcare, personality, support system and life experience. This entire subject, then, is deeply personal, and reflective of the systems we live in.

Here, then, I'm not suggesting an objectively better or worse course of action. I'm letting you know that the solution I present in this book isn't the whole picture. Moving out of old patterns that increase dysregulation and toxic stress is essential to physical and mental health and wellbeing. But it's not the entire solution, and it would be dangerous of me to imply otherwise.

When to work with a practitioner

On page 155, I included an overview of signs you may benefit from working with a trauma trained practitioner. Sheryl Close – a psychotherapist and trauma specialist – shared this perspective as part of a conversation we had while I was researching this book. As well as the general information included in Chapter Four, Sheryl also highlighted some red flags. These red flags indicate that it's highly likely you'll need to work with a practitioner before you move into self-led work. In other words, these aren't mere suggestions, they're highly recommended. Here are some of Sheryl's red-flags that indicate support is needed to achieve regulation and healing:

If the reader is experiencing a chronic health condition like fibromyalgia or chronic dissociation, has no capacity to experience safety, has high levels of intense emotions that fluctuate rapidly or has a cluster of diagnoses like social anxiety and OCD, they'll need additional support and deeper processing before they can implement self-led tools.

Likewise, if the reader has a birth story that was scary for the mother, or they were around stress and dysfunction or experienced medical interventions in their first few years of life, they're likely to need co-regulation before they can self-regulate. Another example would be a lack of memories for certain time periods in their life, because this shows that the brain has been overwhelmed and has not been able to download memories and experiences. Another red flag would be if people are unable to experience happiness, pleasure, satisfaction, contentment or enjoyment in any area of their life.

Someone experiencing any of the above would need a somatic regulation-based modality such as Transforming Touch to bring regulation, capacity and resilience to the nervous system before they do therapeutic or self-led work.

If any of these red flags are relevant to you, self-led work may be challenging. Know that you have not done anything wrong, that it's common, and that choosing support is an expansive, self-led choice that will lead to more expansive, self-led choices over time.

Who to work with

As you take self-led action, it's likely that at some stage you'll want to do deeper therapeutic work to process and release trauma and/or help you co-regulate. If you do, I recommend researching further into the following practices:

- Transforming Touch (TT)
- Somatic Experiencing (SE)
- Internal Family Systems (IFS)
- Eye Movement Desensitisation & Reprocessing (EMDR)
- Hakomi Method
- NeuroAffective Relational Model (NARM)
- Deep Brain Reorienting (DBR)
- Somatic Regulation and Resilience (SRR).

The choice of which treatment modality to use is very personal and highly dependent on what you're experiencing and what you need. For example, if you feel called to more greatly anchor into your adult self and create a sense of separation from your trauma, find an IFS practitioner. If you sense that you need to discharge trauma energy from your body, consider finding an SE practitioner.

As a general principle, I would add that timing is everything with these treatments. EMDR, for example, is a powerful and effective way of processing old beliefs and memories. But if undertaken too early, when there's not enough stability and regulation, the experience can feel overwhelming. Getting some advice on which treatment to use and when can be a very valuable use of your resources. I and my team can offer this advice if you need, so head to my website if you feel you need informed guidance to find the right modality for you.

As a final thought on who to work with, I'd add that what matters most is that the practitioner you're working with feels like a safe place to land. Sadly, many come to my own clinic having had traumatic experiences in sessions with other therapists and practitioners. These therapists were, I suspect, well-meaning, but caused harm because they were not regulated enough and stable enough to 'hold' these clients during challenging moments. The therapists claimed to be trauma-informed, but did not have the personal healing or the professional qualifications to warrant this label.

I say this with a certain amount of hesitancy, because there are many excellent practitioners out there and I do not want to create any sense of fear or threat around this choice. But it would be irresponsible of me not to flag this.

If in doubt, talk to people – ask around. Personal recommendations can be a good way to find like-minded, effective practitioners.

Trauma treatment centres

I've spent the past few weeks mulling over which trauma treatment centres I would *unreservedly* recommend. These kinds of treatment centres are either:

- Intensive Outpatient Programs (IOPs), so you live at home but go into the treatment centre for therapy and treatment.
- Or, they're residential, so you go and live at the facility for anywhere between one week and twelve months.

There are some great facilities doing excellent, innovative work. But I can't recommend them because I don't know where you're at and what you need. What I'd recommend for one client would potentially be very different to what I'd recommend for the next person who walks through the door.

So, what I ask is that if you feel that you or a loved one needs intensive trauma treatment, get in touch with me or ask your own therapist or psychologist to recommend somewhere. As I said at the end of my last book, I'm a real human who wants to help. If you need support and guidance, you can find me at sarahwoodhouse.com or email me at hello@sarahwoodhouse.com.

I dearly hope the self-led approach I've described in this book lights you up and helps you move into deep healing, empowerment and real change.

Appendices

Appendix A

Adverse Childhood Experiences (ACEs)

In a groundbreaking study conducted in 1995 by the Centers for Disease Control and the Kaiser Permanente healthcare organisation in California, ten ACEs were identified.[1] Since then, the term has been expanded to include community events, in recognition that a chronic stress response can be triggered by experiences inside and outside the home.[2]

Original ACEs:

- Emotional, physical or sexual abuse
- Physical or emotional neglect
- Household mental illness
- Household substance abuse
- Exposure to domestic violence
- Parental separation or divorce
- Incarcerated relative.

Expanded ACEs:

- Discrimination
- Chronic poverty
- Violence in the community
- Community disruption
- Poor housing quality and affordability
- Lack of opportunity, economic mobility and social capital.

Appendix B

Imagination techniques

I've included scripts for two mind-body visualisations below, but using guided audios is easier for most. You can find free audios of these visualisations, along with others, at my website: sarahwoodhouse.com

Visualisation One: Safe place

Lie or sit down, get comfortable and close your eyes. Begin to relax and let go of the day. Take deep breaths down into your belly, and as you slowly exhale, release tension from your body.

Now, begin to visualise a place that feels comfortable and nourishing. Picture yourself sitting or lying in the space – build the picture around you. This could be somewhere real – somewhere you've felt safe, regulated and nourished. Or it could be somewhere fictional. For some people it's a sandy beach; for others maybe a book-lined library. All that matters is that this place feels good to you and your body.

Take your time as you build the picture. Surround yourself with things you love, things that feel good to you. What can you hear while you're in this place? Perhaps waves lapping on the shore? Birds? A gentle breeze? A crackling fire? Allow your imagination to create and as it does so, allow your senses to take part – feel, hear, see and smell this safe place. Once you've created your safe place, simply be here, breathing and connecting to it.

When you're ready to leave, start to wiggle your toes and stretch your body. Gently and slowly reconnect to the environment around you. But remember – you can come back as often as you like. It's yours.

Visualisation Two: Healing light

Lie or sit down, get comfortable and close your eyes. Begin to relax and let go of the day. Take deep breaths down into your belly and as you exhale, see if you can release any tension you are holding from your body. If that is not possible, simply notice the tension and allow it to be there.

Move your attention to your heart space. Visualise a golden sphere of energy and light at your centre. Breathe here for a moment, focusing on the sphere and imagining yourself connecting with this strong, powerful central part of yourself.

Now, visualise light flowing gently into your heart space, into and around this golden sphere, bringing energy and compassion into your centre. Breathe here, allowing yourself to take in as much goodness as you need in this moment. Feel the safety and nourishment this light brings – allow it and expand it.

When you're ready, picture this light moving around your body, healing and nourishing you as it moves through you. Take your time with this – picture the light moving into places that need nourishment and healing.

Now, picture your entire nervous system glowing with a calming, beautiful light, as if it's responding to this nourishment. Your entire body is now full of healing light. Breathe here and know all is well – that you're healing.

When you're ready to move out of the visualisation, start to wiggle your toes and stretch your body. Gently and slowly reconnect to the environment around you, perhaps noticing things you can see, hear and feel. But remember – you can come back to this healing light whenever you need to.

Appendix C

Resources for presence and mindfulness
Meditation and Mindfulness
There are a huge number of resources available to help you practice meditation and mindfulness. Here are some that I rate highly:
- Insight Timer (app)
- Tara Brach guided meditations – free audios
  tarabrach.com/guided-meditations/
- Rubin Museum – free audios
  rubinmuseum.org/spiral/mindfulness-meditation/
- Mindfulness – how to
  freemindfulness.org

Yoga Nidra and Non-Sleep Deep Rest (NSDR)
Again, there are many resources available to help you start practising yoga nidra and NSDR. Here are three I use personally:
- For yoga nidra, Ally Boothroyd's YouTube channel has many free audios
  youtube.com/@SarovaraYoga

- For NSDR, Andrew Huberman's website links to various free audios
  hubermanlab.com/nsdr
- Insight Timer (app) has yoga nidra and NSDR audios

Appendix D

Below are lists of the many ways the nervous system's survival response shows up in our mind, behaviour, body and beliefs. It's impossible for me to include every experience. As we move into curiosity about our own experience of fight, flight, freeze, fawn and collapse, we notice the unique subtlety of how these things show up for us. But the lists can be a helpful place to start, as they'll connect your awareness to your own experience. The experiences listed below overlay onto the different states. For example:

- Irritability indicates we're experiencing fight energy.
- Overthinking and adrenalised planning indicate we're experiencing a flight response.
- Overwhelm indicates that we're moving from fight/flight into a freeze response.
- Dissociation and a blank stare indicate that we're moving from freeze into collapse.
- Mental fixation on others indicates that we're, at least partly, in a fawn response.
- Despair and hopelessness coupled with lethargy indicate that we've moved into collapse.

I have not grouped these experiences into the five different survival responses, because there's too much overlap. As I've mentioned before, it's common to experience a sense of flight *and* fawn, or fight *and* freeze. These states are energies – they move and weave into each other.

Mind

- Endangerment thoughts (e.g. 'My son is unsafe')
- Catastrophic thinking (e.g. 'Everything's going wrong')
- Intrusive shocking thoughts
- Hypervigilance (i.e. searching for danger/mistakes)
- Overthinking
- Planning
- Figuring everything out
- Thoughts about running away
- Thoughts about pressing the 'fuck it' button
- Thoughts of not enoughness and failure
- Perfectionism (i.e. 'I must do better' or 'I must do more')
- Worry, rumination and obsessive thinking
- Self-blame and self-hate
- Judgement of self or others
- Criticism of self or others
- Irritability and frustration
- Negative thinking and pessimism
- Thoughts about not being liked/loved
- Confusion
- Brain fog
- Overwhelm
- Mental Paralysis
- Fixation on others' wellbeing
- Fixation on how to repair/be liked
- Thoughts of despair and hopelessness

- Thoughts about giving up
- Suicidal ideation.

Behaviours
- Rushing
- Speeding up
- Compulsive cleaning/tidying
- Overworking
- Eating quickly
- Compulsive scrolling and internet use
- Fidgeting
- Overscheduling
- Skin picking
- Sleep disturbance
- Picking a fight
- Defensive reactions
- Arguing
- Shouting
- Limited self-care (e.g. not taking toilet breaks, showering, resting, going to bed, etc.)
- Avoiding people or places
- Under/overeating
- Rituals around food and eating
- Compulsive exercise
- Compulsive spending
- TV bingeing
- Alcohol and drug use
- Gambling
- Blank stare
- Shutting down
- Isolating
- Sleeping excessively.

Emotions

Humans experience hundreds of different emotions, all stemming from the core ones we're all familiar with: anger, fear, sadness, disgust, surprise and happiness. These primary emotions can be experienced at many different intensities from mild to extreme, such as from annoyance to rage for anger, or from peaceful to ecstatic for joy. The core emotions can also combine to create a new type of emotion. For example, anger combined with disgust can lead to contempt, or happiness combined with trust can lead to love.

Emotions are just different energy patterns moving through the body, which we then interpret and name. Seeing emotions as energy helps us understand that they're supposed to flow and move, and need to be felt and released rather than supressed, ignored or blocked.

To help you widen your emotional vocabulary, here are some of the secondary emotions that stem from the core six:

Anger	Fear	Sadness	Disgust	Surprise	Happiness
Hurt	Anticipation	Disappointment	Disapproval	Startled	Playful
Irritated	Nervous	Lonely	Embarrassed	Confused	Content
Critical	Anxious	Inferior	Ashamed	Amazed	Proud
Frustrated	Insecure	Vulnerable	Appalled	Excited	Powerful
Mad	Scared	Victimised	Awful	Shocked	Curious
Defensive	Panic	Abandoned	Revolted	Dismayed	Loving
Defiance	Terror	Despair	Horrified	Astonished	Thankful
Rage	Dread	Powerless	Loathing	Disillusioned	Optimistic
Injustice	Overwhelm	Hopeless	Revulsion	Awe	Confident

Sensations

The way we experience and name sensations is very personal. There are no right or wrong experiences or words to use to describe them. But it can be helpful to see how others describe their sensations, because hearing the words can connect our awareness to our own bodily sensations. Here are some words my clients commonly use:

Tight	Constricted
Gripping	Tense
Clenched	Holding
Weight	Powerful
Heavy	Achey
Hard	Pressure
Knotted	Sharp
Buzzing	Prickly
Light	Tingly
Fuzzy	Airy
Shaky	Shivery
Warm	Hot
Cold	Numb
Dropping	Sinking
Rushing	Moving up
Big	Small

Traumatic beliefs

These are the final conclusions we can come to about ourselves, other people, relationships and the world following a traumatic experience. There are many, but these are ones I commonly hear clients speak about:

- I don't deserve love.
- I don't deserve happiness.
- I don't deserve success.
- I am a bad person.

- I am worthless.
- I am inadequate.
- I am shameful.
- I am not lovable.
- I am disgusting.
- I am not good enough.
- I cannot cope.
- I am broken.
- I am damaged.
- Other people are unsafe.
- Relationships are unsafe.
- Vulnerability is unsafe.
- Intimacy is unsafe.
- Authenticity is unsafe.
- Other people cannot be trusted.
- Men can't be trusted.
- Women can't be trusted.
- Love is painful.
- People abandon me.
- The world is cruel.
- Life is unfair.
- The world is unpredictable.
- Life is chaotic.
- The world is unsafe.

Appendix E

There are many different ways of naming and categorising values. Brené Brown has compiled a list of values that are specific to her work, however I think it's a great place to start and applicable to all areas of life:

Accountability	Ethics	Kindness
Achievement	Excellence	Knowledge
Adaptability	Fairness	Leadership
Adventure	Faith	Learning
Altruism	Family	Legacy
Ambition	Financial stability	Leisure
Authenticity	Forgiveness	Love
Balance	Freedom	Loyalty
Beauty	Friendship	Making a difference
Being the best	Fun	Nature
Belonging	Future generations	Openness
Career	Generosity	Optimism
Caring	Giving back	Order
Collaboration	Grace	Parenting
Commitment	Gratitude	Patience
Community	Growth	Patriotism
Compassion	Harmony	Peace
Competence	Health	Perseverance
Confidence	Home	Personal fulfillment
Connection	Honesty	Power
Contentment	Hope	Pride
Contribution	Humility	Recognition
Cooperation	Humour	Reliability
Courage	Inclusion	Resourcefulness
Creativity	Independence	Respect
Curiosity	Initiative	Responsibility
Dignity	Integrity	Risk-taking
Diversity	Intuition	Safety
Environment	Job security	Security
Efficiency	Joy	Self-discipline
Equality	Justice	Self-expression

Self-respect	Teamwork	Uniqueness
Serenity	Thrift	Usefulness
Service	Time	Vision
Simplicity	Tradition	Vulnerability
Spirituality	Travel	Wealth
Sportsmanship	Trust	Wellbeing
Stewardship	Truth	Wholeheartedness
Success	Understanding	Wisdom

© 2020 by Brené Brown, LLC, brenebrown.com/resources/ dare-to-lead-list-of-values/

Appendix F

The occipital bone sits the base of your skull. To find this bone, put both your hands on the back of your skull and nod your head slowly forwards. You'll feel the two points of the skull bone as they meet your neck, either side of the spinal column.

Allow your left hand to drop, but keep your right hand on the right occipital bone. Using two fingers, press firmly on the lowest point of the bone, where it meets the neck, and move the skin to the right and then the left. Which direction was there greater resistance? Start where there was the greatest resistance. So, say the resistance was greatest moving the skin to the left, once again move the skin to the left and hold for about 20 seconds. Then, move the skin in the other direction and hold for 20 seconds.

Now, allow your right hand to drop and move your left hand to the left occipital bone. Repeat the steps above on the left hand side.[1]

Resources

If you are experiencing high levels of trauma symptoms and/or PTSD, please contact your local doctor for a treatment referral, or use one of the urgent support phone lines below if you need help now.

Australia

For urgent support, call Lifeline on 13 11 14 for confidential 24/7 counselling and referrals.

UK

For urgent support, call Samaritans on 116 123 for confidential 24/7 support.

USA

For urgent support, please contact National Suicide Prevention Lifeline on 1800 273 TALK.

Notes

Introduction

1. World Health Organization, *ICD-11: International classification of diseases*, (11th revision), 2022.
2. Ibid.
3. Felitti, V.J., Anda, R.F., Nordenberg, D., Williamson, D.F., Spitz, A.M., Edwards, V., Koss, M.P. & Marks, J.S., 'Relationship of childhood abuse and household dysfunction to many of the leading causes of death in adults: The Adverse Childhood Experiences (ACE) Study', *American Journal of Preventive Medicine*, 14(4), pp. 245–58, 1998.
4. Burke Harris, N., *Toxic Childhood Stress: The Legacy of Early Trauma and How to Heal*, Bluebird, 2020.
5. Dube, S.R., Fairweather, D., Pearson, W.S., Felitti, V.J., Anda, R.F. & Croft, J.B., 'Cumulative childhood stress and autoimmune diseases in adults', *Psychosomatic Medicine*, 71(2), pp. 243–50, 2009.
6. National Scientific Council on the Developing Child (2005/2014), *Excessive Stress Disrupts the Architecture of the Developing Brain: Working Paper 3*, updated edition, retrieved from developingchild.harvard.edu
7. Porges, S.W., 'The polyvagal theory: new insights into adaptive reactions of the autonomic nervous system', *Cleveland Clinic Journal of Medicine*, 76 (Suppl 2), S86–90, 2009.
8. Porges, S.W., 'The polyvagal perspective', *Biological Psychology*, 74(2), pp. 116–43, 2006.

9 Dana, D., *Anchored: How To Befriend Your Nervous System Using Polyvagal Theory*, Sounds True, 2021.
10 Hughes, K., Bellis, M.A., Hardcastle, K.A., Sethi, D., Butchart, A., Mikton, C., Jones, L. & Dunne, M.P., 'The effect of multiple adverse childhood experiences on health: a systematic review and meta-analysis', *Lancet Public Health*, 2(8), e356–66, 2017.
11 International Coaching Federation, *2020 ICF Global Coaching Study: Executive Summary*, PricewaterhouseCoopers, 2020.

Chapter 3
1 Walker, P., *Complex PTSD: From surviving to thriving*, Azure Coyote, 2021.
2 Lerner, R., *Living In The Comfort Zone: The Gift of Boundaries in Relationships*, Health Comunications, 1995.
3 Felitti, V. J., Anda, R. F., Nordenberg, D., Williamson, D. F., Spitz, A. M., Edwards, V., Koss, M.P. & Marks, J. S., 'Relationship of childhood abuse and household dysfunction to many of the leading causes of death in adults: The Adverse Childhood Experiences (ACE) Study', *American Journal of Preventive Medicine*, 14(4), pp. 245–58, 1998.
4 Hughes, K., Bellis, M.A., Hardcastle, K.A., Sethi, D., Butchart, A., Mikton, C., Jones, L. & Dunne, M.P., 'The effect of multiple adverse childhood experiences on health: a systematic review and meta-analysis', *Lancet Public Health*, 2(8), e356–66, 2017.
5 Autoimmune issues: Dube, S.R., Fairweather, D., Pearson, W.S., Felitti, V.J., Anda, R.F. & Croft, J.B., 'Cumulative childhood stress and autoimmune diseases in adults', *Psychosomatic Medicine*, 71(2), 2009.
Chronic fatigue: Heim, C., Wagner, D., Maloney, E., Papanicolaou, D.A., Solomon, L., Jones, J.F., Unger, E.R. & Reeves, W.C., 'Early adverse experience and risk for chronic fatigue syndrome: results from a population-based study', *Archives of General Psychiatry*, 63(11), 2006.
Multiple sclerosis: Shaw, M.T., Pawlak, N.O., Frontario, A., Sherman, K., Krupp, L.B. & Charvet, L.E., 'Adverse Childhood Experiences Are Linked to Age of Onset and Reading Recognition in Multiple Sclerosis', *Frontiers in Neurology*, 2017; Pust, G.E.A., Randerath, J., Goetzmann, L., Weierstall, R., Korzinski, M., Gold, S.M., Dettmers, C., Ruettner, B. & Schmidt, R., 'Association of Fatigue Severity With Maladaptive Coping in Multiple Sclerosis: A Data-Driven Psychodynamic Perspective', *Frontiers in Neurology*, 2021.
Psoriasis: Akamine, A.A., Rusch, G.S., Nisihara, R. & Skare, T.L., 'Adverse childhood experiences in patients with psoriasis', *Trends in Psychiatry and Psychotherapy*, 2022 Aug.
Chronic obstructive pulmonary disease (COPD): Anda, R.F., Brown, D.W., Dube, S.R., Bremner, J.D., Felitti, V.J. & Giles, W.H., 'Adverse childhood experiences and chronic obstructive pulmonary disease in adults', *American Journal of Preventive Medicine*, 34(5), pp. 396–403, 2008.

Notes

Migraines: Siego, C.V., Sanchez, S.E., Jimenez, M.L., Rondon, M.B., Williams, M.A., Peterlin, B.L. & Gelaye, B., 'Associations between adverse childhood experiences and migraine among teenage mothers in Peru', *Journal of Psychosomatic Research*, 2021.

Inflammatory Bowel Disease: Gnat, L., Mihajlovic, V., Jones, K. & Tripp, D.A., 'Differentiating Childhood Traumas in Inflammatory Bowel Disease', *Journal of the Canadian Association of Gastroenterology*, pp. 172–8, 2023.

6   National Scientific Council on the Developing Child (2005/2014), *Excessive Stress Disrupts the Architecture of the Developing Brain: Working Paper 3*, updated edition, retrieved from developingchild.harvard.edu

7   Harvard University, Centre on the Developing Child, *Toxic Stress*, 2025, retrived at: developingchild.harvard.edu/key-concept/toxic-stress/

Chapter 4

1   Anderson, F., Schwartz, R. & Sweezy, M., *Internal Family Systems Skills Training Manual: Trauma-Informed Treatment for Anxiety, Depression, PTSD & Substance Abuse*, PESI Publishing & Media, 2017.

2   Shrier, A., *Bad Therapy: Why The Kids Aren't Growing Up*, Swift Press, 2025.

3   Neff, K., *The Elements of Self-Compassion*, 2025, retreived from self-compassion.org/what-is-self-compassion/

4   Ibid.

Chapter 5

1   Lally, P., et al., 'How are habits formed: Modelling habit formation in the real world', *European Journal of Social Psychology*, 6(40), 2009.

2   Wilson et al., 'The Eighty-Five Percent Rule For Optimal Learning', *Nature Communications*, 2019.

Chapter 6

1   Ranganathan, V.K., Siemionow, V., Liu, J.Z., Sahgal, V. & Yue, G.H., 'From mental power to muscle power – gaining strength by using the mind,' *Neuropsychologia*, 42(7), pp. 944–56, 2004.

2   Dispenza, J., *You Are The Placebo: Making Your Mind Matter*, Hay House, 2014.

3   Reddan, M.C., Wager, T.D. & Schiller, D., 'Attenuating Neural Threat Expression with Imagination', *Neuron*, 100 (4), pp. 994–1005, 2018, quoted in *Neuroscience News*, 'Your Brain on Imagination: It's a Lot Like Reality', neurosciencenews.com/imagination-reality-10320/

Chapter 7

1   Silsbee, D., *Presence-Based Coaching: Cultivating Self-Generative Leaders Through Mind, Body and Heart*, Jossey-Bass, 2008.

2   Cass, R., *Polishing The Mirror: How To Live From Your Spiritual Heart*, Sounds True, 2014.

3   Verhaeghen, P., *Presence: How Mindfulness and Meditation Shape Your Brain, Mind, and Life*, Oxford University Press, 2017.

4   Luders, E. et al., 'Global and regional alterations of hippocampal anatomy in long-term meditation practitioners', *Human Brain Mapping*, 34, pp. 3369–75, 2013.

5   Lutz, A. et al., 'Long-term meditators self-induce high-amplitude gamma synchrony during mental practice', *Proceeding of the National Academy of Sciences*, 101, 16369–16373, 2004.

6   Fialoke, S., Tripathi, V., Thakral, S. et al, 'Functional connectivity changes in meditators and novices during yoga nidra practice', *Scientific Reports* 14, 12957, (2024).

7   Huberman, A., *Dr Andrew Huberman's Guide to NSDR*, 2025, retrieved from: hubermanlab.com/nsdr

8   Stankovic, L., 'Transforming trauma: a qualitative feasibility study of integrative restoration (iRest) yoga Nidra on combat-related post-traumatic stress disorder', *International Journal of Yoga Therapy*, (21), pp. 23–37, 2011.

9   Chambers, R., Lo, B.C.Y. & Allen, N.B., 'The Impact of Intensive Mindfulness Training on Attentional Control, Cognitive Style, and Affect', *Cognitive Therapy and Research*, 32, pp. 303–22, 2008.

Chapter 8

1   Schwartz, R., *No Bad Parts: Healing Trauma & Restoring Wholeness with the Internal Family Systems Model*, Ebury, 2023.

2   Ibid.

3   Earley, J., *Self-Therapy: A Step-By-Step Guide to Creating Wholeness and Healing Your Inner Child Using IFS, A New, Cutting-Edge Psychotherapy*, Pattern System Books, 2012.

4   Schwartz, R., *You Are the One You've Been Waiting For: A New Approach to Intimate Relationships with the Internal Family Systems Model*, Vermillion, 2023.

Chapter 9

1   Bandura, A., *Social learning theory*, Prentice-Hall, 1977.

Appendix A

1   Joining Forces For Children, *What Are ACEs?*, 2025, retrieved from joiningforcesforchildren.org/what-are-aces/

2   Milken et al., *The Pair of ACEs Tree*, retrieved from publichealth.gwu.edu/sites/g/files/zaxdzs4586/files/2023-06/resource-description_pair-of-aces-tree.pdf

Appendix F

1   Rosenberg, S., *Accessing the Hidden Power of the Vagus Nerve*, Read How You Want, 2017.

Acknowledgements

Many people have contributed to this book. I wrote the words, but these words were shaped, nipped and tucked through a joyfully collaborative process. In particular I want to thank Brandon VanOver at Penguin Random House Australia and Charlotte Croft at Green Tree. You have wholeheartedly supported and encouraged me while offering your own wisdom and experience whenever it was needed – as all outstanding editors do. Thank you.

Likewise, I'd like to thank Caroline Hewlett, Lizzie Dorney and the PR team at Bloomsbury for helping get the book out into the world. A big thanks to Clive Hebard for your thoughtful final edits too.

As always, I want to thank my literary agents Lisa Moylett and Zoë Apostolides. Thank you for your continued support, and for getting another book across the line. I greatly appreciate you both. Thank you.

I also want to thank the clinicians and practitioners who shared their time and wisdom with me. Sat Dharam Kaur, Dane Ensley, Ingrid Clayton, Julia Samuel, Sheryl Close, Lou Lebentz, Brad Reedy, Josh Dickson and Calum Morrison – thank you. You have added something important and beautiful here. I'm grateful that you trusted me and my work enough to allow yourself to be woven into these pages.

Finally, I'd like to end on a heartfelt thank you to the researchers and practitioners whose work and theories have fed into this book. To Dr Stephen Porges, Deb Dana, Richard Schwartz, Dr Peter Levine, Dr Gabor Maté and Dr Kristin Neff: thank you. Your work has provided a spring-board for this book. You are woven into these pages, and I'm sincerely grateful for your contributions to the field of trauma healing.

Admittedly, the humans I'm about to list did not shape, nip and tuck the words themselves, but they supported and loved me through the process of writing. So, thank you, from the top:

Roo, Fern & Wren – for your patience and support. You have made more space for my work and purpose than most children are asked to do. I recognise this, appreciate this and understand the impact it has. I deeply appreciate you. More than this, I am in awe of all three of you. Although my work has taken up precious space in your life, I dearly hope that it also inspires you to trust yourself in a world that will often try to convince you not to.

Mum & Dad – for your unconditional love. Your capacity to accept me and the path I chose for myself means everything to me. You are exceptional parents. If there were awards, you'd get one. I am so very grateful for you both. Thank you.

Sally Harrington – for always believing in me. Your love for me is like no other other I've ever experienced. I increasingly understand that what we have is what love *is*: unconditional, fierce, gentle, spacious, respectful, deep and seamlessly able to see and hold every single part of each other. Thanks also for the dark, inappropriately timed suicide jokes. These also fit into my idea of what love is. See you on the other side . . . right? Don't you f**king dare.

Ian Dunt – for your loyalty and wisdom. Yes, I called you wise. I also know you well enough to understand that I will deeply regret this choice of words as they are repeated back to me to prove your rightness over the next decade. The sadness of this relationship is that I can't even add an exclamation mark to let anyone who may read this understand that I am joking. Oh, the grammatical bind. You've helped me navigate an exceptionally difficult time with love, patience and perspective. Thank you for everything. To still choose each other all these decades later is a testament to just how much love there is.

Simon Reed – for supporting me through this year with a seemingly unshakeable belief in me. Your willingness to share your experience and adult perspective, but also (and often in the same sentence) your capacity for irreverence and humour, has made all the difference. Thank you for making me smile every day since I was last but definitely not late, and for showing me how incredible life can be when we show up real and authentic. Thank you for trusting me and for showing me, every day, that I can trust you. Mainly though, thank you for suggesting coffee . . .

Laura Bailey – for your love, support and endless pragmatism. I think it's highly likely you're the strongest woman I know. You help me be better in more ways than I'm able to articulate. Thank you.

Neil Woodhouse – thank you for making space for this book in the midst of a difficult year and for telling me all those years ago that I could and should write my first book. You are a remarkable man and I hope 'all this' leads to the happiness you deserve.

Nova Maxwell – for your acceptance, love and steady presence in my life. To still be standing by each other all these years later means so very much to me.

Katherine Chandler – you are an incredibly capable human being. I don't think it's a stretch to say that I wouldn't have a business were you not by my side. Thank you for your support, patience, enthusiasm and incredible capacity to get the job done.

Also by Sarah Woodhouse

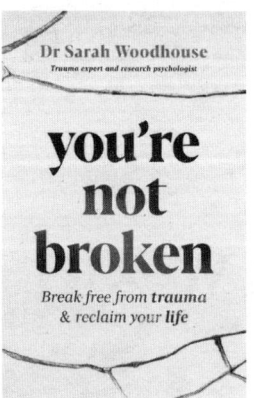

Trauma can manifest as anxiety, shame, low self-esteem, over-eating, under-eating, addiction, depression, confusion, people-pleasing, under-earning, low mood, negative thinking, social anxiety, anger, brain fog and more.

Traumas, big or 'little', leave us trapped in cycles of dysfunctional behaviours, negative thoughts and difficult feelings. Yet many people are unaware they're stuck in old reactions and patterns that stem from their past traumas. Many of us are wary of the word and push it away instead of moving towards it and learning how to break free.

In *You're Not Broken* Sarah Woodhouse teaches you what a trauma is and how to recognise when, why and how your past is holding you back. She gently explains the pitfalls of ignoring awkward, upsetting episodes and how true freedom comes from looking back at your past with honesty. Then, sharing the latest research-based techniques and her own personal experience, she guides you towards breaking the trauma loop, reawakening your true self and reclaiming your future.

sarah woodhouse

An invitation...

If you feel called to work with me, please get in touch.
You can find out more about how we can work
together on my website: sarahwoodhouse.com

My website also holds all the free resources I've
mentioned in the book – the audios, tools and
principles that will help support your
self-healing journey.

You can sign-up to my free newsletter,
Notes On Freedom, here too.

If you have any questions, or just need to touch base,
you can email me at hello@sarahwoodhouse.com

With love and respect,

S. x